A Spouse's Intimate Alzheimer's Journal

Deeper Than Blue

MY HUSBAND'S ALZHEIMER'S JOURNEY

Other Titles by

AMANDA G.

Fiction

Arms of the Magnolia

Beyond the Fire

Confliction

Deeper
Than
Blue

MY HUSBAND'S
ALZHEIMER'S JOURNEY

AMANDA G.

GW Publishing LLC

For information about this title or to order other books and/or electronic media, contact the publisher:

GW Publishing LLC
gwpublishingllc.com

Cover and interior design by The Book Cover Whisperer:
OpenBookDesign.biz

978-1-7367268-2-2 Paperback

Printed in the United States of America

FIRST EDITION

FOR MY HUSBAND

CONTENTS

Acknowledgments..i

Chapter 1: THE PURGE...1

Chapter 2: I SAW THE SIGNS.....................................6

Chapter 3: SOLDIER 10

Chapter 4: TAKE ME TO THE WATER 13

Chapter 5: THIS MASQUERADE................................17

Chapter 6: HELP 20

Chapter 7: SOMEBODY'S WATCHING YOU 23

Chapter 8: OLD SCHOOL REMEDY 29

Chapter 9: GOING THROUGH................................. 33

Chapter 10: THE ADVOCATE 38

Chapter 11: IN THE MIDNIGHT HOUR 44

Chapter 12: HIGHER GROUND 47

Chapter 13: VOGUEING IN THE ER............................ 52

Chapter 14: NO VISITORS ALLOWED 54

Chapter 15: SOUND OF SILENCE 58

Chapter 16: AFTER THE FALL................................. 66

Chapter 17: A BLAZING GRACE............................... 70

Chapter 18: APPETITE FOR ALZHEIMER'S 73

Chapter 19: BLENDER SPLENDOR 78

Chapter 20: FEAR OF HOPE 83

Chapter 21: LEANIN' 90

Chapter 22: FICKLE WILL FLEE................................ 96

Chapter 23: LIGHT AT THE END 102

Chapter 24: DEEPER THAN BLUE............................. 105

Chapter 25: WHAT THE END'S GON' BE 108

APPENDIX A... 111

About the Author 119

Deeper

Than

Blue

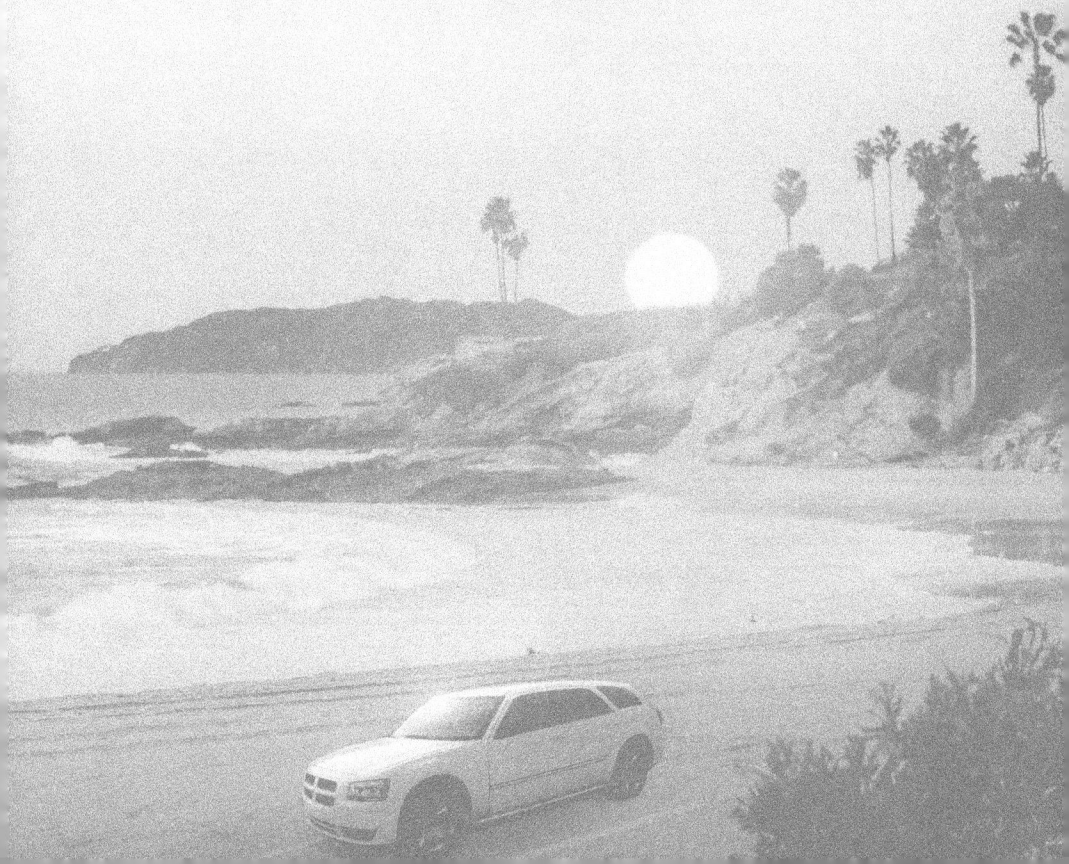

ACKNOWLEDGMENTS

THIS STORY COULD NOT BE TOLD without acknowledging the support, professionalism and love showered on my husband, MH, and me during my husband's journey through Alzheimer's. Whenever there was a need, want or an unuttered cry the right people magically appeared.

I call them angels in our midst-women and men doing their jobs with an added dose of sensitivity. I thank and praise the doctors, nurses, and caregivers who took the time to listen when I was riddled with anxiety and fear.

I praise the spiritual connectors who prayed with us when we were battle-weary.

I thank my dear friends and family who read early drafts of the manuscript and provided invaluable comments. Thank you for encouraging me to share my very personal story with the world.

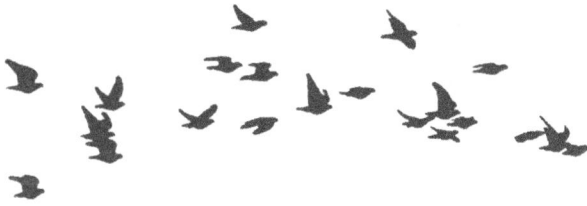

CHAPTER 1

THE PURGE

I was terrified but not surprised when my husband joined the ranks of almost seven million Americans living with Alzheimer's. Through the trickle of years, I recognized MH's subtle, then radical personality changes-repetitive storytelling, lack of interest in current topics and deep dive into keeping secrets about the smallest thing.

In 2016 The diagnosis dropped like a death sentence on MH's legal career. Naturally, this proud and highly competent attorney rebelled. "I outperform ninety-five percent of the lawyers in my office," he correctly asserted. But the risk was too high. I had visions that one day, amid brilliant courtroom oratory, sneaky plaques and tangles strangling his brain would leave him speechless before a judge.

My family history made me painfully aware of the havoc that dementia and its subcategories of illnesses, including Alzheimer's, wreak on a family. My mother lived with dementia for several years before passing away at age ninety-one. My father died from Alzheimer's complications at age eighty-six.

The progression of each family member's disease was radically different. One common element tied them together. The "Stare", that confounding blank expression, emanating deep within the soul, ushered my loved ones down a path of no return.

It was no coincidence when a representative from the Orange County, California Alzheimer's Association spoke at a networking luncheon shortly after my husband's diagnosis. With great trepidation and in hushed tones I approached the speaker at the end of Q & A. Was I embarrassed or reluctant to admit that life had dealt us a blow that we could not dodge? Determined to confront the monster stalking our lives, I scheduled a meeting at the Alzheimer's Association. My husband was not onboard.

In the parking lot of the Alzheimer's Association building, I begged MH to hold my hand and walk with me on this journey. MH's feet dug in like a bull's. My obstinate husband ignored my pleas to follow me inside. Angry eyes bounced around his defiant face. His lips were drawn into an uncharacteristic scowl. MH wanted no part of hearing more bad news.

Tears scorched my eyes. I folded my lips to keep from screaming. Ten minutes of patient negotiations escalated into subtle threats. *I can't take care of you, if you shut me out.* Ultimately, MH relented. Heavy feet scraped the ground as we entered the building.

Our representative, Adrian, could not have been more sensitive. Her father, a prominent attorney in Orange County, California (like my husband) fought valiantly against his diagnosis. For months after being diagnosed Adrian's father insisted on continuing to work. In Adrian's opinion, it was not about money. It was the battle of a proud man to maintain dignity and independence.

"And your father. How is he now?" MH interjected his first comment during the session.

"He died two years ago. Right after his eightieth birthday."

"So, there's no cure for Alzheimer's," MH asked. He already knew the answer.

"Not at this time."

Air whooshed out of the room.

"There are drugs that can slow the progression. Talk to your doctor about that. Our job is to educate people, raise funds to find more treatments and hopefully a cure."

In 2023 a new drug, Leqembi, was announced. The drug was touted as effective in slowing progression of the disease in cases of early-stage Alzheimer's. Leqembi was an amazing breakthrough for millions who had recently been or will be diagnosed in the future. The bad news was that the drug arrived too late for my husband who had progressed to a later stage.

I asked myself, would MH have taken Leqembi if his Alzheimer's was in an earlier stage? Possibly not. He resisted taking Aricept and subsequently Namenda, prescribed after his diagnosis. I counted his pills when a bottle remained full after it should have been empty. When I questioned whether he was taking his meds, his only answer was the Stare.

My husband plunged deep into self-help and so-called natural remedies without evidence that any such remedies would cure or alleviate his symptoms. When I saw traces of blood in his stool, I became alarmed, rushed him to Urgent Care. Thankfully, there was no sign of internal bleeding.

The Costco sized bottle of turmeric in his blossoming natural remedies collection (the "Stash") looked suspicious. I confiscated the turmeric. The bleeding stopped almost immediately.

As a proponent of holistic healing, I did not resist his chosen path, except when he went overboard, like overdosing on turmeric. If one capsule is good, try three, he might have reasoned. My instinct about turmeric turned out to be spot on. Turmeric is a blood thinner that can cause negative side effects for people taking other blood thinners. My husband was taking Coumadin for blood clots. Turmeric plus Coumadin was not a good match. MH had not researched possible side effects before leaping right in. It was up to me, his primary caregiver, to pull him out of the deep end.

My vow, "To love and to cherish, in sickness and in health," I took seriously. But I was shut out, forced to become a sleuth in my own home. I closely monitored MH's prescription medications and the Stash, which was not easy. The Stash was concealed in odd places: in dusty recesses of his closet, pockets of unused suit jackets, and dark corners of the guest bathroom vanity. One good thing resulted from my vigilance. I was compelled to clean spaces that would not normally be reached.

Purging closets and cabinets became an excellent source of distraction. It gave me something to do when there was nothing to do about the underlying source of my husband's illness. I spent hours checking prescription labels and discarding expired medications. I donated lightly worn clothing (his and mine) to charities that support men and women re-entering the work force.

Self-help books and magazines overcrowded our mailbox daily. For Alzheimer's patients, false prophets and fake remedies abound. The Internet was a swamp, MH's cell phone a breeding ground for credit card fraud. Several times I closed or disputed accounts when unscrupulous people had gotten the best of him. MH was always good about paying his bills. He now lacked the insight to distinguish between legitimate bills and outright fraud. A colossal burden fell on me to draw the line between his right to use debit and credit cards and the obligation to shield MH from the ugly side of the world. Slowly, I whittled down his use of bank cards until he operated on a cash only basis.

Our roles evolved. I was no longer just his wife. I was his protector.

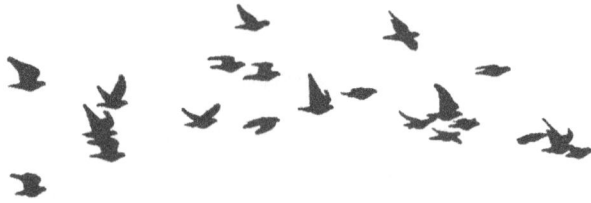

CHAPTER 2

I SAW THE SIGNS

Our family questioned if I was "losing it" when I suggested my husband was "losing it" long before he was formally diagnosed with Alzheimer's. Suspicion was in their eyes, not on their tongues. "Wait", they pushed back. I had waited almost four years before allowing my concerns to be uttered to close family.

At my son's law school graduation, an event steeped in pomp and circumstance, my usually friendly husband crawled into a shell. MH spent long spells staring into the great beyond.

I had grown accustomed to compensating for his lapses, filling in sentences, physically ordering his steps when his sense of direction failed him.

It was convenient to attribute the sudden personality change to stress-the stress of his job as a public defender overwhelmed by hundreds of cases. His performance impacted the freedom, life, or death of other human beings. Stress of a weekend warrior whose muscles were not twitching like they used to when he jogged for miles or biked over two hundred miles with three amigos. MH was so good and passionate about his job that when the fog rolled in, he carried on without missing a beat. Or so it seemed until the threads of life unspooled.

Articulate, outgoing and dependable were characteristics frequently attributed to my husband. Then the dreaded disease hijacked his personality, turning him into a distant stranger. Repetitive discourse practiced in his mind substituted for true conversation. If I asked about events of the day, politics, culture, or history (his favorite subject) he stared blankly. It was mind-boggling, coming from a man who previously had opinions about everything.

Consumed by pressure to keep the house and our respective law practices in order, I lost sight of how far MH had drifted. I was between the proverbial rock and a hard place, needing to know, but not sure if I wanted to know what hit him. I was losing the one that I had known, loved, and been married to for forty-one years at the time of MH's diagnosis.

I blundered around the Internet, researching Alzheimer's, depression, mid-life crisis and withdrawal from family and friends. I wanted to rule out Alzheimer's as a possibility.

Armed with my degree from Google University, I bogarted into an appointment with his primary physician. I showed up in the parking lot of the doctor's office. MH's dead eyes startled with alarm. "What are *you* doing here?" MH demanded. I kept stepping. His arm barred the door.

"Last night you said it was okay for me to meet you here."

"Well, it's not okay. Go home."

"I know you're afraid, but we can deal with this. I'm here to help."

"You're not coming into my appointment," he snapped.

I threw up my hands. "Okay. I'll just sit in the lobby and wait until you come out."

His unsteady shuffle preceded me up the stairs. It had been years since his hip replacement. According to MH, his orthopedic surgeon found no medical explanation for the obvious deterioration in his ability to walk. Or maybe the surgeon had offered an explanation that MH refused to share. Of late his medical history was a closely guarded secret. He had become a privacy junkie, lying, or intentionally omitting essential facts.

At the far end of the waiting room, MH ignored me. He avoided eye contact when the doctor's assistant summoned him to the exam room. He made a wide arc around me, like garbage to be avoided. The door closed behind him. I whipped out my cell phone and texted his sister in D.C. Several minutes later she called back. "He's not letting you in. Says he has a right to privacy." My heart sank. If she could not get through to him, no one could.

I slipped a note to the doctor's receptionist. "Please deliver this to the doctor while he is examining my husband. It's important."

Dr. Swan was not surprised to receive my note. I had done everything I could, including asking questions about MH during my annual check-up, to make Dr. Swan aware that I was alarmed by my husband's mental and physical decline. Dr. Swan did not take the bait. He informed me that unless MH gave permission, he could not talk to me. The doctor was correct, but I was determined to get to the root of our problem. Maintaining the status quo was not an option.

Throughout much of our marriage, our days began with early morning walks. One morning the pace was brisk, but not the least bit challenging for MH, the cyclist and swimming enthusiast. His pace slowed to a turtle's crawl. As he fell further behind, I turned, walked back to him, and said, "See what happens when you drink beer before bedtime," I chuckled.

"Shut up bitch." His mean, aggressive response almost knocked me off my feet. My soul shattered into a million jagged pieces. MH had never thrown profanity at me, not even during serious arguments. I did not know this man. His gentle demeanor was what initially attracted me to him.

I clenched my tears and accelerated my steps. "You'll never walk with me again." Little did I know the truth of my prophecy.

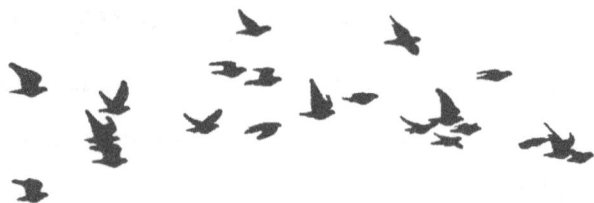

CHAPTER 3

SOLDIER

When Dr. Swan uttered the words, "Let your wife in," I entered the battle that, according to the experts, we would not win. The half-hearted, unenthusiastic participation of my partner made the odds even worse. It was clear from the beginning. MH did not want to know what was happening to him.

On a referral from Dr. Swan, I made an appointment with a neurologist, Dr. Pooni. To MH's dismay, I had taken responsibility for scheduling and making sure he attended important appointments. MH had astutely avoided keeping the appointments he feared might lead to discovery of the true nature of his illness. I hooked arms with MH, grousing and swearing under his breath, and babied him into Dr. Pooni's exam room.

Dr. Pooni was young, new to the profession. She maintained her distance from the patient, physically and emotionally.

MH pulled out the oldest trick in his playbook. "Are you old enough to play with that thing?" he asked, pointing to the stethoscope.

Dr. Pooni's focused, searing coal eyes and forced scowl thwarted him. MH shrank in his seat. His bottom lip protruded into a pout.

From an oversized manila envelope Dr. Pooni pulled black and white film, indisputable evidence of irreversible damage to MH's brain.

"Sir, you have Alzheimer's." She plunged the dagger in. No foreplay, no "I'm sorry." My head reeled. I could not imagine what was going through MH's mind. I reached for his hand. His fingers refused to curl around mine. He was frozen, unwilling to claim the bad news.

"We did an MRI of the brain with and without contrast. It showed significant atrophy of the anterior temporal lobes," Dr. Pooni continued. "The frontal lobes showed significant brain shrinkage. "

I stammered. "So, what does this mean? He's still working, driving around, like everything is everything."

"Your husband must make adjustments in his life. First, quit lawyering. Don't drive unless accompanied by another driver. Avoid the freeway. Stay on city streets."

MH cut her a fisheye that should have brought the doctor to

her knees. Doctor Doomsday rocked on. "And by all means, don't make any financial decisions."

He reacted as if she sentenced him to life in prison. I sensed MH strategizing, making escape plans.

The diagnosis was numbing, but not surprising. My Google research had reached the proper conclusion years earlier. Every day I prayed that my conclusion was wrong. The coldness with which the doctor delivered the diagnosis shuddered me to the bone. I wanted to crawl beneath a weighted blanket and hide.

Neither MH nor I could absorb the inconvenient truth. Alzheimer's steered our lives down a rushing, unfamiliar river. He or we might capsize.

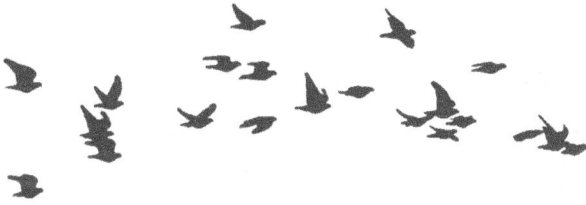

CHAPTER 4

TAKE ME TO THE WATER

Five grueling years had passed since MH's formal diagnosis. By the grace of God, he was able to stay at home during those years until the weight literally overpowered me.

One evening I arrived home, exhausted from a rough day at work, and found MH stuck on the soiled couch, unable to stand, rollover or drop to his knees. I tossed my purse and briefcase on a chair and lunged into leveraging position. He was dead weight. MH could not follow basic directions or assist me in the least. We had always been able to find a "work around" for this type of predicament. I ran outside to the shed and found a walker my mother had used when she lived with us. I posted the walker in front of him. He groused, "I'm not using that thing." Frustrated and exhausted,

I snapped, "Use it or I will have to call the fire department." That got his attention.

The next morning, before my visit to the chiropractor (I pulled a muscle freeing MH from the couch) I came to grips with the fact that I could no longer handle my husband alone or allow him to be home alone, not even an hour.

The diagnosis compelled dizzying adjustments in our home life. I hired a string of part time in-home caregivers and drivers to assist him with bathing, grooming and transportation. He fought every attempt to provide support until he could no longer function by himself.

For years I pretended that the skirmishes over getting him into the shower were no big deal. I developed a scheme. The driver hired to take him to his favorite places was not allowed to take him out unless they confirmed that MH had showered. We were not asking for daily dipping, just maintenance of basic hygiene. It broke my heart to see MH morph from a meticulous, well-groomed, best dressed man in the courtroom, to a person afraid of water. This was puzzling. Prior to the "no water phase" he spent hours in the pool every day even in cold weather. What was worse? Fighting over staggering six-hundred-dollar gas bills (from MH heating the entire pool for hours and conveniently forgetting to turn off the heater) or forcing anti-aqua man to wade in shower water occasionally.

I approached his resistance to bathing totally wrong. Instead of using coercion I should have researched the psychological and physiological causes of his resistance. My husband showed signs of depression from being unable to make minor and major decisions about his own life. It had to be humiliating having his wife cajole him into taking a shower or checking behind him to see if the washcloth was wet after he came out. The embarrassment of having me or an outside caregiver monitoring his bathing habits had to be profound.

The master bedroom of our home had an old, sunken Roman style tub with a deep step down. The tile was slippery and unsightly. My husband's condition gave me incentive to push forward on a bathroom remodel that I had contemplated for years. I got rid of the Roman tub, created a level walk-in shower without a lip or ledge to step over. I purchased new, fluffy towels and aroma therapy vials. I ushered my husband into our new space, complete with a shower chair. MH took one look, did a U-turn and walked out. I would be the only one to take advantage of this pricey bathroom re-model.

There is no guaranty that any further adjustments (e.g. pre-heating the bathroom for half an hour, playing soft music, being more patient in coaxing him into the bathroom) would have worked. Other adjustments were made, but not on a sustained basis. I felt a sense of failure, failure of patience, which I did not master until much further down the line.

It felt strange, having conversations with other primary caregivers about resistance to bathing. Our shared experiences often ended in comparing caregiving to raising an ornery child. What we learned was that resistance was not just a matter of stubbornness. Our loved ones had experienced actual brain damage. MH's doctor explained, "A child's brain is in the process of developing, expanding. The brain of an Alzheimer's patient is in the process of shrinking."

Once I developed a different perspective, I was able to step back from the triggering incident. Do not take it personally, I reminded myself. I accepted that MH lacked the ability to change annoying habits. The one who had to change was me.

As the battle of "Water Who" receded, new challenges cropped up to take its place. In retrospect that battle was minor compared to the challenges that lay ahead.

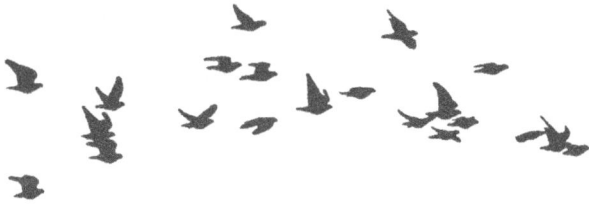

CHAPTER 5

THIS MASQUERADE

My husband was an expert at masking his disease. In the summer of 2019, we visited my son and his family in Dallas. We met for lunch at the Dallas Museum of Modern Art. The temperature was in the high nineties, humidity at its peak. Our feet pounded steamy pavement up a slight incline. I saw MH struggling, so I reached for his arm. Two hip replacements and the battle raging in his mind had him walking like a drunk. He shrugged me off.

Inside the museum there was an exhibit of vintage designer clothing. I got excited about the exhibit. I was the only one. The consensus was that we should eat first then see how we were doing on time. MH insisted on having a glass of wine despite my protest. Halfway through the meal MH's head began to bob. With one arm I grabbed him and with the other pushed away his wine glass. His swoon did not deter him from snatching back the wine glass. Through slurred, garbled speech he demanded, "Leave me alone". My son circled the table to steady him. My daughter-in-law ran for the car parked two blocks away.

At Baylor University Hospital emergency room, they registered MH as a possible stroke victim. He received attention fast. In the fifteen-minute dash to Baylor MH's speech had improved substantially.

"Let's get the hell outta here," MH repeated a hundred times while we awaited the results of CT scan, EKG, and blood tests. Two hours later an amiable neurologist, Dr. Douglas, wearing a red and white striped bow tie, breezed in.

"I can tell you're a man of good character," MH cheerily greeted him. "I wear bow ties to court most of the time. The judges love it."

"You're a lawyer, sir?"

"That's correct. And I apologize for wasting your time. A few sips of wine at lunch made me dizzy. I should have known better. Texas heat, in the summer, can wear you out. My grandparents have a one-hundred-acre farm east of here. Sulphur Springs. Ever hear of it?"

And thus began the bullshit. Not the story about the farm, which was true. MH had memorized the amazing history of his grandparents, one generation removed from slavery, yet able to prosper in the segregated South by acquiring land. It was a beautiful story repeated for every stranger that MH encountered. He wove the story into conversation no matter the listener, the place or time. Dr. Douglas patiently waited and listened without interruption.

MH finally took a breath. The bamboozled doctor interjected, "If this man has Alzheimer's, he is the smartest Alzheimer's patient I have ever met."

My eyes rolled to the ceiling. Dr. Douglas promised to send test results, smiled at his new best friend, and patted MH on the back on his way out.

"Let's get the hell outta here," MH badgered the second the door clicked shut.

Four years later when the sound of silence rolled in, I scarcely believed this episode myself. I thought MH would talk forever, keep repeating the same stories until there was no breath. I was wrong.

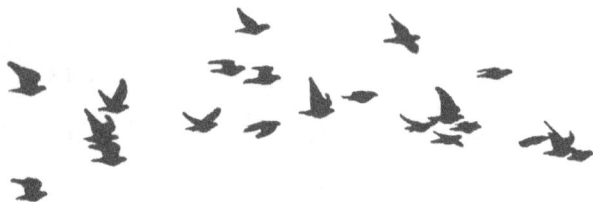

CHAPTER 6

HELP

Doctors were understandably cautious in restricting MH's driving freedom. They did not want to run afoul of my husband, a lawyer trained in DMV defense. I was desperate, privately pleading with his doctors to help me. I hand-delivered a note to MH's latest primary care physician.

"PRIVILEGED AND CONFIDENTIAL
August 27, 2019
Dear Dr. XXXXXX:
Enclosed is the paperwork from my husband's emergency room visit to Baylor University Medical Center in Dallas, Texas. We rushed him to Baylor because he exhibited stroke symptoms while we were

having lunch. His speech became incoherent, he could not smile, his behavior was belligerent, and he had trouble walking. Our son and his wife were present when the incident occurred. Approximately fifteen minutes after the onset of symptoms, the symptoms began to subside. We spent several hours at Baylor undergoing various tests, including CT scan, EKG and blood tests. At the end of the day, he was diagnosed with TIA but no stroke.

What I am most concerned about is that MH has experienced over several years various episodes in which he fainted or nearly fainted, sweated profusely, vomited, or lost control of bladder functions. Afterwards he does not remember the episode or denies that it ever happened. A common thread in the episodes is use of alcohol and warm weather. Even modest alcohol use can be a problem. For example, he had only consumed one-half glass of wine when the incident occurred on 8/20/19.

I have strongly urged him not to drink or alternatively never to drive after drinking, but he ignores my pleas. Just yesterday I noticed that he was out driving after drinking wine. I am at my wits end trying to protect my strong-willed husband. A prior neurologist informed the DMV of his dementia after I spoke to her. DMV tested his driving ability and allowed him to maintain his license. Mechanically, he is a good driver, but the risk is that an episode, seizure, or TIA might occur while he is driving, leading to disaster. I want to avoid injury to him and to others.

I understand your need to protect the doctor/patient privilege, but I have run out of options. Please speak to my husband about the danger of drinking and driving, especially in his condition. He does not listen to me. Any help you provide is greatly appreciated.

Sincerely,

XXXXXXXX"

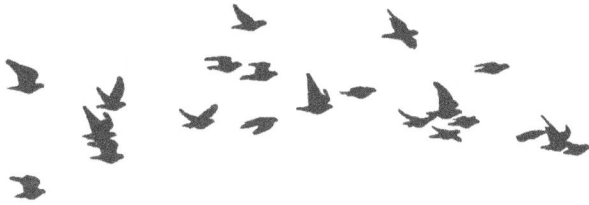

CHAPTER 7

SOMEBODY'S

WATCHING YOU

I thought I had hit rock bottom, but there was more to come. On November 10, 2019 a towering, buff Black police officer (a novelty in Orange County) knocked on our door. Without thinking I, wearing a tattered robe and a doo rag on my head, snatched open the door. The officer introduced himself by a foreign sounding last name that I proceeded to mispronounce.

"Just call me Officer "Q". Is your husband at home?"

"Why do you ask?"

A woman had reported him for harassing her while she walked around the man-made lake near our home.

"What did he say to her?"

Officer Q's answer was vague mumbo jumbo.

I filled in the blanks. "He probably said that he likes the way she walks to his music. He says that all the time."

One thing saved my politically incorrect, Alzheimer's stricken husband from getting arrested. His comments were usually made within the confines of his car, a 2006 Dodge Magnum with ample dings and dents and twenty-two-inch chrome rims. The Dodge with its wide, low riding seats was his world. Frequently, we drove him to Laguna Beach or local parks where MH sat for long stretches of time watching people and cars pass by. He often commented that people within his field of vision were walking or running in sync with Doo Wop music wafting from the Dodge's CD player. When he drove alone the music boomed at vibrating decibels.

His prized collection of well-worn CDs consisted primarily of Doo Wop, late 1950's and early 1960's music (any song by Frankie Lymon and the Teenagers, the Platters, Love Potion Number 9 and Witch Doctor). We had a boatload of CD's at our home, but Oldies were the only thing he wanted to hear. A few exceptions were made for early Motown hits like Smokey Robinson and The Miracles singing "Mickey's Monkey". The same songs or albums played repeatedly. I thought my head would explode.

On a good day his shoulders hunched to the beat. "Mickey's Monkey" sent his shoulders bouncing with glee. If I inserted the wrong CD, he hit eject immediately. Young folks will not remember CD players in cars. They won't recall the CD skipping if scratched, worn out, or if you hit a bump in the road. MH did not mind the interruptions, the nerve grinding skips. Control over his music was all that mattered. Radio be damned.

If the car was parked, he earnestly believed that other cars were driving to "Stayin' Alive" by the Bee Gees. Some days he insisted that cars had faces resembling people or animals. On occasion I was sucked in by the vivid images he painted. "That car looks like Rosie, Stephanie's daughter." I did a double take, had to check myself.

On top of all his other issues MH had a serious hearing problem. Studies have found a correlation between Alzheimer's and hearing loss. They do not suggest that hearing loss causes Alzheimer's. Rather hearing loss increases the risk of Alzheimer's. Missing the sound of a siren or failing to understand a police officer's instructions could have landed MH in the hospital or worse.

I was frustrated daily by the inability to capture MH's attention. Diminished hearing was a major problem for MH long before he was diagnosed with Alzheimer's. By his late fifties the problem reached the point where he could not hear my voice from another room. Unless we were face to face in the same room all communication was lost. He grew impatient, snapped if I attempted to communicate with him in a normal voice. The burden was on me to position myself so he could essentially "lip read".

MH burned through multiple expensive sets of hearing aids. He allegedly *lost* the hearing aids that tested his vanity, then quit wearing replacements "cold turkey". Despite pleas to try again, MH insisted that distorted sound from the hearing aids was worse than not hearing. I threw in the towel.

MH sauntered to the door, grinning at Office Q as if he was welcome company. Gibberish about music, people and cars erupted from my husband's mouth. MH broke the cardinal rule of a good defense attorney. Keep your mouth shut.

I interceded. "My husband has Alzheimer's. I try to keep him from driving, but at this point I can't prevent it. Maybe you can help me with DMV?" Officer Q did not appear inclined to help.

"If he's ever out of line, other than speaking to someone, let me know."

The officer responded, "I've had my eye on him for a while."

"Has he done anything wrong?"

"No, he just makes people nervous."

"I get it. Black man, cruising, playing loud music in Orange County. What next? "I retorted sarcastically.

"Keep an eye on him." Officer Q turned to leave.

My blood pressure shot up. Was he shaming me for not doing enough? "I am doing the best I can. Alzheimer's is not a crime." I spoke to Officer Q's back.

An hour later I opened one side of my garage door to take out the trash. There was a forty something White stranger lurking in the driveway and peeking inside the garage. Startled, I asked, "Can I help you?"

"That car." He pointed to MH's Dodge Magnum. "The man driving it. Does he live here?"

"Who are you?"

"A concerned father. He's been driving around our neighborhood, harassing my teenage kids."

My heart sank. I knew exactly where MH had been. There was a large condominium complex a couple of miles from the house that he loved to drive past. I knew it because he always wanted to drive through whenever I chauffeured him. The place was not particularly interesting. But there was something about row after row of beige buildings with white trim that fascinated him.

"What did he do?"

"Staring at my kids. This wasn't the first time. He drives past, real slow, like he might do something."

Here we go again, I thought. "I am sorry if your kids were intimidated. My husband is ill. Alzheimer's. He is harmless."

The stranger said, "Oh," and turned to walk away.

"How did you find our house? Did you follow him here?" He did not answer. I started to worry. Is he a neighborhood vigilante? Does he have a gun under his jacket? What if he had shot my husband, former army officer, former corporate attorney, officer of the court, a man with no history of violence? I would be another Black widow on TV, standing teary eyed beside Benjamin Crump.

The next day I called MH's primary physician and recounted both incidents. The doctor referred MH to a second neurologist who ordered another round of tests, including a mobile three-day EKG.

It was the longest three days of my life. My husband was a shorter, chocolate version of Frankenstein. His head was completely wrapped in gauze and bandages. Multi-colored wires, attached to leads on his hairy chest. A bulky monitor protruded from his pocket. The stares and whispers of onlookers did not faze him one bit.

Our neighbor saw MH at the grocery store and phoned to snoop. "Did your husband have brain surgery?"

I had to laugh to keep from crying. I knew immediately, I could not wait for the doctors to get on the same page or for the DMV to pull his license. Someway, somehow, I had to stop MH from driving.

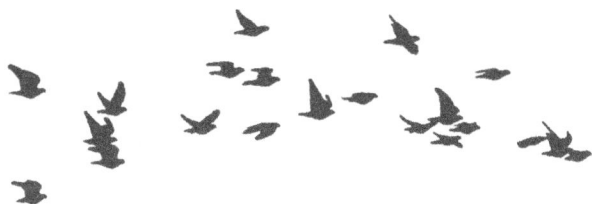

CHAPTER 8

OLD SCHOOL REMEDY

I lived in constant dread that Alzheimer's would grab hold of my husband while he was behind the wheel. I had visions of MH suddenly losing his sense of direction, stopping on the freeway, oblivious to where he was. I could see him barreling into a five-year old pedestrian, catching a case of wrongful death that would land us in poverty.

Dr. Pooni had tried to curtail his driving. She notified DMV, which she was professionally required to do, of my husband's Alzheimer's diagnosis. MH was livid. He saw it as an encroachment on his freedom. DMV summoned MH to take a driving test, which he passed with flying colors. Driving, his specialty, had not been noticeably impacted. Not yet.

The owner of the caregiver placement agency arrived at 8 a.m. on a Monday morning. I was familiar with working through agencies because of my experience with my mother. Her care needs were quite different from his. She was physically debilitated. He was still on his feet, ambulatory although visibly slower as months rolled on. At that time MH was sharp enough to circumvent attempts to hide his keys. Several times he called AAA to replace his keys after I hid them. I called AAA's front office, begged them not to come to our home to replace keys. Each time the AAA operator agreed. Each time MH called, AAA dispatched a technician who made a brand new, expensive set of keys to the Dodge. I contemplated stringing the duplicate keys on a chain to symbolize my wasted investment in AAA.

I came up with an idea. I hired a caregiver/driver to keep MH company on his trips through the neighborhood. Two hours a day, five days a week he was chauffeured in the gas guzzling Dodge. On Saturdays and Sundays, I drove him around.

MH's thirst to wander alone by car was not quenched. At the end of the caregiver's shift, before I got home from work, MH hit the streets with renewed vigor.

After explaining my predicament to the owner of the caregiving agency, he popped the trunk on his Cadillac Seville. He handed me something I had not seen in years. Lo-Jack, an old school heavy metal lock for the steering wheel, disabled the car when the lock was properly engaged.

MH's response was unexpectedly mild. "Get that thing off my car," he said when he first laid eyes on Lo-Jack.

"No can do. The whole purpose of hiring the driver was to give you the pleasure of riding around without hurting yourself or somebody else. The neurologist told you not to drive alone. But you're still doing it. I had no choice but to lock the car."

He seemed to accept my answer. Too easily.

Next morning, stepping out of the shower, a bad feeling washed over me. I dashed to the garage. The driver's side door to the Dodge was wide open. Armed with a hammer, saw and chisel, MH did battle with Lo-Jack. He chipped away specks of paint, left ragged scratches on the steering wheel. Lo-Jack stood its ground.

Victory lasted less than twenty-four hours. "Where are you?" I screamed into the phone on day three of our Lo-Jack adventure. The Dodge was missing from the garage. I had failed to take the key out of the lock.

"Just looking around," he answered nonchalantly. He did not know that I had put a tracker on his phone. It felt awful invading his privacy. Never during our long marriage had I snooped into his business, even when there was probable cause. I refused to live my life worrying about a grown man. This was different. There was too much at stake. His life, liberty, and our financial future. I did not want the cops at my front door again. I did not welcome confrontation with a neighborhood vigilante, armed or unarmed.

I turned on the tracker, got in my car and proceeded to the

same condominium complex where he liked to "look around". Look around at what, I asked myself as I cruised through the land of beige condos. There was absolutely nothing of interest, except in his mind.

I rolled up behind MH and leaned on my horn. In his rearview mirror startled eyes locked with mine. He stepped on the gas, drove in circles for fifteen minutes with me trailing behind. At a stop light I pulled up next to the Dodge, rolled down my window and begged him, "Please go home."

"I'm going to McDonald's," he insisted and sped off. Now I was angry with myself. Lo-Jack, a marvelous low tech life saver invented to prevent car theft, only worked if used properly. I deserved to be anxiously sitting in the parking lot of McDonald's waiting for my vacant eyed husband to order the same breakfast he ordered every day for two years. Breakfast burrito, senior coffee with two Splendas and two creams inside, two ketchups, one salt, one pepper, and one stirring stick.

Under the Golden Arches this negligent, frazzled wife almost burst into tears. Instead, I laughed to keep from crying.

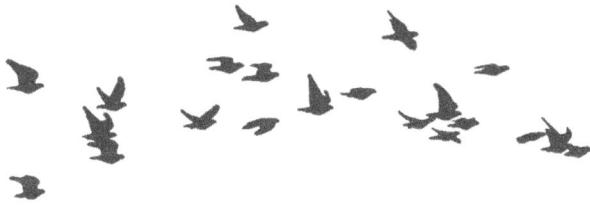

CHAPTER 9

GOING THROUGH

It began as a peaceful Sunday morning walk with gospel music streaming from my earbuds. The call came from a caregiver at the board and care home where I placed MH five years after the diagnosis. The caregiver had found MH on the floor sitting on top of his right leg.

The caregiver described MH's condition as awake, but unresponsive when paramedics quizzed him. His face was frozen. He spoke no words. The left lower lip drooped. Paramedics feared a stroke.

On my race to ER I was petrified. Less than a year earlier my car sprinted the same path to the same hospital where my ninety-one-year-old mother lay dying. A massive stroke, the latest among many, had landed her in the hospital a month earlier. The stroke left her unable to speak or swallow. The prognosis was dire. Doctors, hospice workers, everyone had told me it was a matter of time. Still, I assumed she would recover. She always had.

In a flashback a swarm of paramedics encamped around my mother, pulse barely perceptible, breathing feeble puffs of life. They worked feverishly to save her. I knew from the paleness of her skin, the looseness of her limbs that she was on the last of her nine lives. I remembered intense ringing in my ears, lost perception of time. For a brief, unforgettable moment Mama's eyes locked with mine. Don't torture me, her eyes pleaded. She was done.

I touched the paramedic's arm, pumping her fragile chest, and whispered, "Let her go." Mama's eyes looked homeward as she answered the trumpet of God.

Paramedics and hospital staff faded away. I held my mother's hand, lay my head upon her breast one last time. A final kiss. An impossible goodbye.

I snapped out of it, needed to concentrate to find a space in the congested ER parking lot. Where did all these people come from early on a Sunday morning? I circled twice, exited to a side street, found a space at the far end of the overflow lot.

I sailed through the doors of ER. My nerves were shot. I waited in line for a visitor's badge. Waited for the receptionist to locate my husband's bed. Reminded myself to breathe or risk passing out.

MH's bemused look, his smile substitute since Alzheimer's went on the rampage, stretched across his face. I kissed his forehead and reassured him that everything was okay. He mumbled words. I wept. His speech, though garbled, was coming back. I settled in to wait for results from the CT scan that would determine if MH had had a stroke.

Hours into my wait Doctor Liu breezed in. "The good news is that the CT scan is negative. Your husband did not have a stroke." Relieved, I grabbed Dr. Liu's hand and shook it, casting aside COVID protocol and the fact that Dr. Liu did not give off a touchy, feely vibe.

My elation was short lived. "I am more concerned about the leg wound," Dr. Liu continued. "It looks bad."

"What leg wound? This is the first I've heard of it," I responded.

The doctor snatched back the lightweight hospital blanket. A third of MH's right leg was covered with ruptured blisters. Someone had taken a potato peeler and removed the top layer of his skin or so it seemed

Into a rabbit hole of doctor speak I spiraled. His creatine kinase count was off the chain. "What is creatine kinase?" I asked, feeling stupid.

Dr. Liu opined, "It could be caused by infection in his brain, muscle or heart. But I don't think that's what it is. More likely, it's Compartment Syndrome." The name was quirky, difficult to remember. The symptoms would have resounding impact. By evening MH's right leg was the size of a tree trunk. The skin stretched taut, shiny, ready to pop.

MH's fall and prolonged lack of circulation led to a dangerous condition. To alleviate pressure, an emergency fasciotomy was performed. For those blessed to never have experienced it, fasciotomy is a surgical procedure where fascia is cut to relieve pressure stemming from loss of circulation. The urgency of relieving the pressure was intense. If the tension or pressure was not relieved, the result could have been loss of limb. Amputation.

My first encounter with two large, uncovered wounds occurred when I returned from the cafeteria. The wound care nurse, calmly removing layers of gauze, chirped about the seriousness of the wounds. I took one look, backed up against the wall and spun into the hallway. My stomach roiled. I searched for a barf bag, just in case.

I was blown away by what I had seen. On his outer leg was a ten-inch-long incision, flayed open like a side of beef. The inner leg incision was shorter, but deeper. Red muscles and white tendons bulged out.

"What the hell," I moaned into my KN95 mask. Right then I knew, there was a long, tedious road ahead. I prayed for my husband, too out of it to appreciate the complexity of what he faced. I took several deep breaths to calm my racing heart and reentered my husband's room.

"Why are the wounds open? Why didn't they stitch him up." I asked the nurse.

"The wounds must heal from the inside. Over time, the wounds will close by themselves."

MH's leg was attached to a wound vacuum whose job was to suck out the blood and mucous to help the wound heal. I could not count the hours spent watching the see-through container fill with what I called wound muck. Wound care nurses measured the muck, then dumped it when the container filled.

Measurement was also taken of his urine, collected through a Foley catheter (stuck inside his penis) and captured in a see-through urinal hung on the side of the bed. The urine changed colors daily. Over a two-week period, the urine changed from cranberry red to mustard yellow to light amber signifying that the antibiotic drip was slowly working against infection and the stubborn virus, Sepsis.

Wounds weeping, bodily fluids oozing, monitors beeping, MH seemed distant from the pain. It seemed that his mind had disconnected from his body.

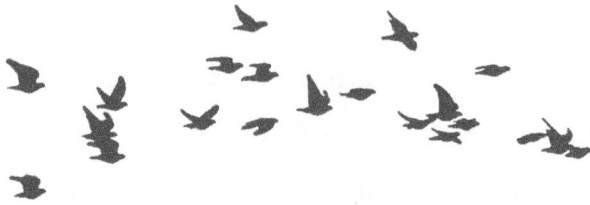

CHAPTER 10

THE ADVOCATE

Two weeks after admission MH was released from the hospital back to his board and care home. A great deal of thought and discussion went into whether to send him to a skilled nursing facility as an interim step or directly back to the board and care.

I advocated strongly for the board and care. Every day, multiple times a day during his hospital stay MH begged "Get me out of here. Take me back to where I was before." He never called the board and care "home", but it was his comfort zone. A place where they cleaned him, fed him, and picked him up when he was stuck on his bed or in a chair. Sometimes he got stuck, standing up, not knowing where to turn.

Hard decisions had to be made before discharge. Could the

board and care handle him, given his continuing need for antibiotics and wound care? The flurry of activity was sometimes overwhelming. I settled my mind, attacked each problem as it came. Too often there were five or six issues cropping up in one day. Rather than focusing on "woe is he or woe is me", I transcended into a state of constant gratitude, thanking the Creator for giving me the strength to stand by my husband.

As his advocate I listened to what my husband had to say. "Listening" consisted primarily of gauging his emotions through touch and feel, studying his puppy sad eyes and facial expressions for clues. MH rarely communicated with the hospital staff. They asked him a question. He lay there, mute. If he spoke when I entered the room, they would be startled that he talked at all.

Silence grew louder and longer each day. Aphasia, defined by The American Heritage Dictionary as "Partial or total loss of the ability to articulate ideas in any form, resulting from brain damage," went into overdrive during his hospital stay. I noticed the change in his speech right away. I attributed the decline of his verbal ability to his recent trauma, tried to convince myself that once he was "home" and healed, his speech would come back.

"This man," I told the nurse's assistant who cheered when MH spoke my name, "was a skilled defense lawyer, has a B.A. in speech, delivered impassioned messages at our church, was revered for his oratorical skills."

My voice, protective and combative, fought for his reputation and dignity. Was it not enough to fight one battle at a time? For loved ones of Alzheimer's patients, the hardest thing to accept is that the person, as we know them, is never coming back.

I listened intently to the case managers who patiently explained the benefits of a skilled nursing facility as an interim step. MH's wounds required constant attention. If an infection developed and went untreated, it could cost him his leg. I had already dismissed amputation as an option. My husband, in his obviously depressed state, could not handle it. I also knew that exposure to a new, sterile environment would quickly kill him off. It was a balancing act, the battle of the mind versus the body. It was hard to see my way clearly in this lose/lose contest.

I was warned by the experts to temper my expectations. I remembered the story told by Adrian at the Alzheimer's Association. Her father, the retired attorney, had believed, to the day that he breathed his last breath, that he would be the exception, the one who out distances The Big A.

Dr. Pooni had shown us MRI images, side by side of MH's brain versus a "normal" brain. MH's brain looked as if a two-year-old had been let loose with crayons, drawing squiggles outside the lines. Was I in denial about my husband's prognosis or properly balancing considerations of MH as the patient and MH the man?

This time I was better prepared for my job as an advocate. My experience with my mother taught me a lot. First, I could not be passive as decisions were made. Knowledge was power and I had to acquire that knowledge *while simultaneously dealing with my loved one's illness on a daily, hourly basis.*

I learned not to wait until it was time for him to be released. Early on, I established a relationship with the case manager(s). The assigned case manager was subject to change on any given day. I researched the skilled nursing facilities available through MH's health plan. I read positive and negative reviews on each available facility.

I recalled how my mother's medical plan had provided me the name of the skilled nursing facility where my mother was being transferred *on the same day scheduled for transfer.* I raced through the streets, pulling together the equipment and clothing she needed upon discharge. I called my dear cousin, begging for help. "Do me a favor. Go online and check out this skilled nursing facility. I just found out. They're transferring Mama today. It's a newer facility in an upscale neighborhood. Looks beautiful in the pictures. But check it out just to be safe."

Minutes later my cousin called back screaming, "Hell to the no! That place is a death pit. Not one positive review. Auntie can't go there."

I put my foot down at the hospital (Note that this hospital was different from the one where my husband was being treated). I refused to allow my mother to be transferred until we found a better skilled nursing facility. Contrary to what hospital personnel would have had me believe, they could not force me to accept the first option presented. I understood the hospital's need to move patients out to make room for newer, at-risk patients. The hospital was not a hotel. Reluctantly, the hospital informed me of my right to appeal the decision. The appeal, which I dreaded, would buy Mama some time. All I wanted was a space in a place where my mother could recuperate in peace.

During the two days it took to find an acceptable skilled nursing facility the tension in my mother's room radiated off the walls. Mama ended up in a larger, urban facility. It was not the fanciest, but the staff was kind, and they had a good program for rehabilitation. On the downside, the facility was a forty-minute drive from my office without traffic. There was always traffic in the suburbs of L.A.

I learned from my mother's experience that each health plan maintained its own list of available skilled nursing facilities. Just because Joe raved about his stay in a spa like rehab facility, did not mean that facility was available to my loved one. The skilled nursing facility had the ability to accept or reject a patient for any number of reasons, including overcrowding or the inability to meet the patient's needs.

It worked in MH's favor that the number one and number two skilled nursing facilities on my vetted list declined to accept MH due to his recent bout with Sepsis. My strong recommendation to transfer MH back to the board and care became the only viable option.

Decisions were made rapidly in the hospital. I was not shy about asking to speak to a doctor. Not being fluent in "doctor speak" did not deter me. If I did not understand what was being said, I asked the doctor or nurse to break it down into layman's terms. Sometimes the nurses' approach was more digestible. Nurses tended to spend more time with the patient. I made my meetings or phone conversations more productive by researching subject matter that confused me. For example, I had never heard of the term "compartment syndrome" until the surgeon who performed the fasciotomy on my husband explained it to me. After his very detailed description I went home and looked it up. My research did not qualify me as an expert by any means, but it allowed me to better understand why the surgery was necessary in the first place.

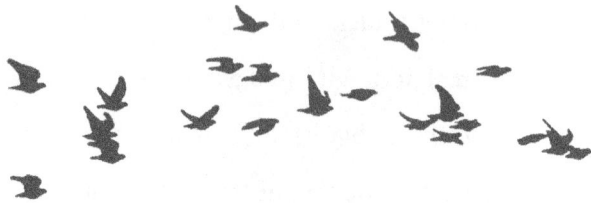

CHAPTER 11

IN THE MIDNIGHT HOUR

"Unhook me or kill me," the patient screamed from stall twenty-three in the emergency room. It was our second trip to ER in less than two weeks. Hours into the ER ordeal we waited for MH to be assigned a hospital bed. Loaded down with recyclable bags carrying water and snacks, a lightweight hoodie and hours of stored up anxiety, getting sprung from ER sounded like the Promised Land. My discomfort paled in comparison to my husband's. MH was too geeked up to sleep, disoriented by the unfamiliar environment, and the glaring lights beaming down on him.

MH's largest weeping wound had turned angry, red with bacteria. I blamed myself for steering him back to the board and care.

If Miss-Know-It-All (me) had pushed to send him to the skilled nursing facility, maybe this relapse could have been avoided.

After a stable, two-week reprieve in the board and care MH grew listless, fever filled and anxious. The in-home wound care nurse did not like what she saw. Neither did I. Back to the hospital we went.

I worried that the germs and viruses flooding the ER on this frantic evening would reach out and grab us. Other patients witnessing the bloody gauze loosely wrapped around my husband's swollen leg, phlegm rattling in his chest, bass cough shuddering his entire body and the putrid, sulfuric odor of his loose stool were probably more afraid of us than we were of them.

No walls or doors separated the parade of human misery. A thin curtain, painted with autumn leaves and only partially covering the opening, was frequently snatched back and forth on a metal rod. A parade of nurses and assistants flowed in and out, taking vitals and attempting to draw MH's blood that clotted with every needle prick.

Directly across from MH's room a wiry Latinx woman cursed at the top of congested lungs. "Dios Mio. What the f.. .k is happening to me? I go to Denny's for a bite of food... I'm too sick to eat, too tired to throw up."

Nana in the bed against the far wall was not too tired. She spewed copious blood, populated with cottage cheesy matter, into a gray plastic tub.

Dios Mio. I thought I would pass out. So, I concentrated on the Phillips Intellivue monitor hooked up to MH and emitting frequent alarms. Heart rate is 126. Blood pressure 171/74. I thought that was good. Turned out it was not. I was too busy preventing MH from yanking out I.V.'s to delve into his blood pressure or dwell on monitor readings fluctuating erratically.

I restrained MH's hands with mine. The strength that he lacked minutes earlier rebounded. He rolled out a secret weapon-spitting like a snuff pinching pitcher on the mound. I bobbed and weaved out of the line of fire, warned ER staff to beware of incoming liquid projectiles.

Fifteen hours from the time he entered ER MH was moved to a different section on the same floor. Suddenly, we had side walls. Although completely open across the front, the walls provided an artificial sense of privacy and safety. We still heard the sounds, moans, coughing and wheezing. It was definitely an upgrade, a splinter of hope that we would soon move to higher ground.

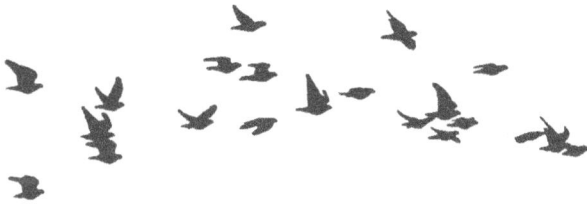

CHAPTER 12

HIGHER GROUND

Before a bank of staff elevators, a transporter applied brakes to the gurney carrying MH to higher ground.

Cindy, a perky ER nurse accompanied us to the new room. MH looked up at Cindy and spoke his first words to someone other than me since our arrival. "Take off that mask. I want to see your face," MH instructed Cindy. Before I could conjure yet another apology for his behavior Cindy complied. MH studied her carefully. "You're a beautiful woman." The green-eyed brunette with major eyelash inserts blushed and giggled. The transporter roared.

I chuckled, "He hasn't lost his ability to flirt". A major consequence of MH's disease was a loss of social filter. My husband said out loud whatever came into his mind. If he saw a fat man, he pointed his finger and loudly proclaimed, "Look at that fat man." If a woman with a big, shapely butt crossed his path, he not only commented on her big butt, but would stare her down until the big butt was out of sight.

Settled into his single occupant hospital room, MH got crazy busy. He pulled the oxygen tube from his nose and snatched the I.V. (inserted with the help of an ultrasound machine due to the difficulty of drawing his blood) from his arm.

The nurse and her assistant strategized about preventing MH from yanking out the IV. Mittens that looked like oversized oven gloves were placed on his hands. Clown accessories. I breathed a sigh of relief too soon. MH began chewing on the Velcro securing the mittens.

He found words to say, "Take these off." Guardian of the gloves, I put them on each time he pulled them off. Explaining to an Alzheimer's patient that we were helping and not hurting him, was an exercise in futility. I stood over his bed, policing busy hands, hoping he would get tired before I did.

Keeping the IV in place was critical after test results rolled in. MH's condition required a steady, high dose infusion of antibiotics. He had ESBL, a more aggressive virus than the Sepsis he acquired during the first hospital stay.

A red quarantine sticker was posted conspicuously at the entrance to his room. More germs circulated in my husband's hospital room than in the Wuhan lab.

Anyone entering his room had to wear blue disposable gloves and don a yellow paper gown. All I needed was a Ukrainian flag to start a parade. Looking like Big Bird traipsing on a cloud, I was busted tiptoeing to the nurse's station. I could not walk down the hall without ripping off the gown and gloves and suiting up anew upon my return.

The paper gown was stiff and surprisingly warm. Long stretches with nothing to do but acknowledge the staff entering and exiting my husband's room left time to imagine how I would redesign the gown. The gown would open from the front with two levels of Velcro to accommodate different sized bodies. I would use softer, more flexible paper. I hated that crunching rustling sound. Don't steal my design idea! I claim a pauper's patent right now.

Keeping track of the tests MH had undergone made me woozy. Multiple CT scans, EKG's, urine and sputum cultures. His bone marrow was suppressed, not churning out red blood cells. CT scan of the chest ruled out pneumonia. Finally, there was a malady that MH did not have. Still, the tests did not explain why during our midnight vigil in ER MH spewed blood like a fountain. I was curious why no one had noted that fact on his chart. Then again, there was so much blood circulating in the ER that night it looked like a knife fight.

"Can he get a sedative?" I pleaded with RN Pamela. "If there is a two for one special, bring it on." I half-jokingly added. Nurse Pamela was not amused. Exhausted from playing Whack A Mole with MH's octopus' hands for over an hour, I made a mental note to bring my own sedative next time.

Hospitalization for an Alzheimer's patient was no fun for anyone, especially the patient. It took an hour for one pill to arrive at my husband's bedside. Based on experience with my mother and stories from other patients, one hour was quite reasonable.

MH had a lot going on: Alzheimer's, virus raging in his blood stream, antibiotics (Ivance) dripping twenty-four seven, a wound vac sucking blood and yellow goo from his leg, and recurring blood clots that heightened the risk from every pill, every procedure.

I sympathized with doctors, nurses and supporting staff who handled the chaos. They were in a pressure cooker. If I turned up the heat too high, hospital staff could slow down their response when I needed them most. That one-hour pill delivery could turn into a three-hour delay. My only recourse would be to trounce through the corridors in my Big Bird costume, waiting to be tackled by security guards.

I opted for the kinder, gentler approach. Calmly, I asked the doctor on duty to explore the cause of the blood that MH spurted while in ER. I offered cell phone photos of MH's blood-stained sheets, pillows, and the blood speckled floor. The doctor graciously declined to receive the evidence.

Almost a week into his second hospital stay and after polite begging by MH's beleaguered wife (me) an endoscopy was ordered.

I remember distinctly the day the procedure was done. The

day before Thanksgiving our trek from MH's room to the G.I. (gastrointestinal) wing began. It felt like a mission to Mars. We exited the center of hospital energy and travelled to a remote wing of the facility. The emptiness of space, the eerie quiet was reminiscent of the opening scene in a horror movie. No one in their right mind signed up for a procedure so close to a major holiday. That is how MH squeezed into their schedule.

My husband was wheeled past patient cubicles with open curtains. Attached to breathing machines, curled in fetal positions, patients with tubes down their throats could not cry out, bug the staff or push alarms for attention. Not a visitor was stirring.

I counted our blessings. No matter how harrowing MH's circumstances, it could have been worse.

There was no waiting room in the G.I. ward. A nurse stationed me in the recovery room lined with rows of empty beds. I resisted the urge to pull out my cell phone and swipe left incessantly. It was time to be still, focus on what I had observed. During MH's short procedure, I prayed for the unknown patients languishing in the G.I. wing. I prayed that they be comforted. I thanked the Master for my husband of forty plus years. But for the grace of God...

The news was good. There was no sign of bleeding in his throat, chest, or belly. The diagnosis: esophagitis, an irritated esophagus causing bleeding and excessive acid reflux. It was treatable.

I gave thanks for the victory, focused on the present and vowed to let tomorrow take care of itself.

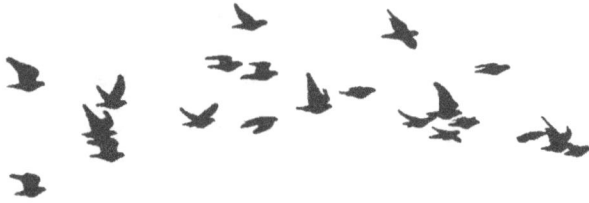

CHAPTER 13

VOGUEING IN THE ER

I could write a whole book on how to gear up for ER. In the interest of time, here are my key takeaways:

1. Wear the heaviest jacket that the weather allows. Nothing fancy. You never know who or what was in the seat before you arrived.

2. Dress in layers. It is usually cold in ER. When you graduate to the upper floors, the temperature may shift radically.

3. Wear rubber soled shoes. There are lots of liquids on hospital floors. Not all of it is water.

4. Wear flexible, stretchy fabrics. These fabrics make sleeping in a chair or curling up on a back breaking bench more tolerable. Spandex is your friend.

5. Bring water and snacks that can be consumed, preferably outside during a quick break. Most hospitals have cafeterias, but they are not all-night diners. I grew rather fond of the soup at MH's hospital. Do not tell them. They will raise prices!

6. Wear a mask. Many hospitals still require masks, despite changes in Covid protocol.

7. That Big Bird suit is a "Must Have", coveted fashion accessory, for a hellish night in ER like ours.

Footnote: The ER scenes described above took place in a suburban, well-equipped, well-staffed hospital. In a different setting, you might get little or substantially reduced service.

No matter the location, ER is a battleground. You never know what will hit you.

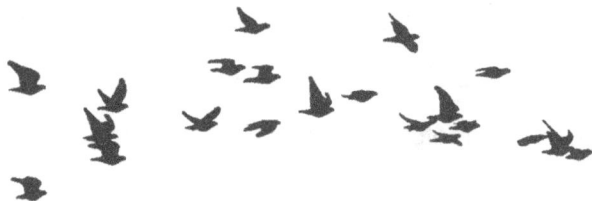

CHAPTER 14

NO VISITORS ALLOWED

One of the gray areas in dealing with Alzheimer's is deciding whether visitors are helpful or harmful to your loved one with the Big A.

First, there are certain courtesies that should always be observed. Drop-in visits are not welcome. People with Alzheimer's develop coping mechanisms. Regularity of their schedule is one way of maintaining control. People who pop in and pester them, "Man, I know you remember me," or "What about that time we did so and so," place a burden upon an Alzheimer's patient to dig for memories that are gone. This is embarrassing to the patient and the caregiver.

Last week I ran into a friend, Gladys, that I had not seen in years.

She and her husband were members at my old gym. I had taken my husband to a doctor's appointment that took way too long. In an uncomfortable wheelchair MH complained repeatedly, "Get me out of here". Gladys glided past, absorbed in her own thoughts. I was slow in recognizing her.

A few minutes passed. Gladys circled back. I called out to her. We hugged. Extreme tension hardened her back. Gladys sat next to me and unloaded an incredible story. Her husband, a muscular, articulate man was also diagnosed with Alzheimer's. She was at the clinic searching for a new doctor for him.

Days later Gladys followed through on our vow to keep in touch. She was overwhelmed, clearly in need to talk to someone who understood her plight. Her biggest concern: Well-meaning people wanted to visit her husband who was a prominent leader in the community before the Big A took control of his life.

Gladys felt guilty saying "no". Alzheimer's had twisted her husband's personality, causing violent outbursts where none existed before. The question loomed, would this once proud, highly intelligent man want to be seen under current circumstances, inside a lock down facility where his freedom was tightly controlled.

"You have a right to say "no", I reassured Gladys. Sometimes an outsider's presence can do more harm than good. If doing good, and not being a lookey-loo, is your goal, offer to take the caregiver out to lunch. Put together a memory book of the good times you spent with the Alzheimer's patient. If you are close enough to the family and have the patience of Job, offer a block of hours to the primary caregiver to give them respite from their duties.

Always check with the primary caregiver before showing up. If you have not been in recent contact with the patient, verify with the primary caregiver that the patient welcomes visitors. Ask if it is advisable to take the patient for an outing and if so, are any special preparations required. In the beginning of his Alzheimer's journey my husband begged everyone (including caregivers, nurses, therapists, housekeepers, family and friends) he encountered, "Take me for a ride."

Before taking the patient away from his home or facility, determine in advance how long the outing may last. Incontinence may be an issue that must be addressed in advance. Eating or drinking should also be addressed to avoid putting the patient at risk of choking.

Be flexible. If you show up for a visit at the appointed time and the patient is not having a good day, reschedule, don't whine. There are many circumstances where a short visit within the home or facility is best for all.

Determine the types of activities the patient enjoys. If going to a restaurant, sitting still and holding a conversation are no longer pleasing to the patient, do not force it on them.

Do not feel offended if the primary caregiver says "no" to a visit. Things may be happening on a physical or mental basis that make a visit ill-advised. For a period of two months MH was in the hospital more than he was out. When he was stable enough to be released, in-home medical care visits consumed MH's days. Physical therapy, occupational therapy, wound care nurses, visits to the primary care physician and the wound doctor were difficult to manage. Calls flooded my phone from various departments of the hospital. It reached the point where I had to keep a separate calendar to remember who was doing what. Filling prescriptions, regulating medication, making sure MH was eating, making sure I was eating kept me on my toes. There was no room for non-essential visits.

Be kind. Call first.

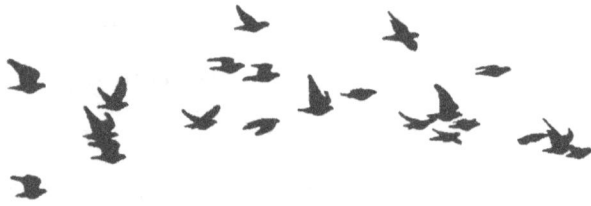

CHAPTER 15

SOUND OF SILENCE

After the fall, the fasciotomy, two extended hospitalizations and multiple debriding of wounds (removal of dead skin), the sound of silence became my greatest fear. I had chafed when his repeated demands ("Get me out of here") bombarded me each time I entered his hospital room. Now his voice, demanding or otherwise, was all I wanted to hear.

MH had gone from fully verbal, to speaking in short, simple sentences, to barely speaking at all. On days when he said one or two words (after extreme prompting) the caregivers and I would literally stand up and cheer.

His verbal expressions dwindled daily, including conversations with me. In a chirpy voice I pleaded with him to greet me, to "Say hi," each time I entered his room. Two-way communication barely existed, except with his torching, melancholy eyes. On bad days, or if I mentioned something that triggered a memory, frown lines gathered around the clouds in his eyes. Sometimes he cried.

He cried, not necessarily out of sadness, but because his heart had been stirred.

What puzzled me most was the inconsistency in his ability to speak. Some days he approached a near normal level of comprehension and articulation. Delays in his responses were minimal, indicating clarity of thought. On his birthday I phoned his sister so that she could wish him "Happy Birthday". He answered every question, including telling her how old he was.

Most days his mind searched for answers. His lips moved without making an audible sound. I learned to wait, be patient for seconds or even minutes to give his mind a chance to catch up.

Trauma had hurled MH deeper into the Alzheimer's Abyss. For years he held some symptoms at bay, by memorizing scripts and exercising maniacally to keep himself in the game. Now he was stripped of all façades, left sitting alone behind the curtain, completely revealed.

My heart crumbled into aluminum sadness that could not be smoothed. I was not allowed to cry. He was watching, always watching, searching the reservoir of my heart.

I dreaded revisiting the article I read months earlier, "Stages of Dementia" written by Compass. The article contained a "Functional

Assessment Staging Tool (F.A.S.T scale)". A rating of 1 on the scale indicated early-stage Alzheimer's. A 7 rating denoted the end stage of the disease. I reluctantly reviewed symptoms of each stage and confirmed what I suspected. My husband's Alzheimer's had fast forwarded into the later stages. In my layman's opinion MH had blasted into stage 6 and flirted dangerously close to stage 7.

Despite all the medical consultations over several years, the F.A.S.T scale was my first clear understanding of where my husband stood. Doctors tended to "beat around the bush" or avoid direct answers when I questioned how far the disease had progressed. Maybe to avoid liability issues. Perhaps they did not really know. They did not see the desperate look in MH's eyes while struggling to identify a thing or person achingly familiar. They missed his flash of anger at my attempts to ban him from behind the wheel.

MH's bed became a sea of pillows, propping up legs that had lost communication with his brain. My fervent prayer, that he would regain some measure of pre-fall mobility went unanswered as days rolled into months and months rolled into a year. His once beefy legs withered over a period of several months into twisted vines that lay motionless.

A year lying on his back, waiting for wicked wounds to heal, reduced MH to wheelchair status.

The march toward the wheelchair began before the events (hereafter called the "Incident") that mowed him down. Summer before the Incident I took him for frequent rides in the Dodge. He complained about walking (using a walker) less than twenty feet from the car to the front door of the board and care. Each time I pulled into the driveway he insisted that the caregiver bring out a wheelchair. At first, I resisted, urging him to walk as much as possible. Ultimately, making it to the door became a bridge too far for a man whose brain was injured. I yielded to reality, called for the wheelchair.

Inside the care home he still used the walker. The progression from walking unassisted to using the cane to using a walker moved at warp speed. It was a matter of weeks between each stage. He resisted every step of the way.

"I'm not using that thing," he insisted, pointing to the walker when the cane failed to provide enough support. Three months earlier "that thing" was the basic black utilitarian wood cane that had "old man" written all over it. One day I surprised him with a gold metal cane with tiny stars that sparkled. He fancied the gold cane, which had been used by my mother when she was alive. I caught him test driving it a few times.

I rustled around my shed and found the gold cane hidden in a nest of cobwebs. I cleaned up the gold cane and delivered it to him the next day. Problem temporarily solved; vanity assuaged.

I understood the need to stroke one's ego once I joined the sixty-five and older clan. Getting old was inevitable. Looking old was reserved for someone else.

A doctor friend had warned that once the patient settled into a wheelchair you cannot get them out. She was right. I felt the battle raging between his body and mind. My husband wanted to walk more than anything. Watching the grimace on his face, his muscles tremble and collapse as he pushed the walker less than two inches was painful. I hummed marching songs to give him a beat to step to. His mind refused to cooperate. Scraping cruel hot pavement, his feet refused to lift an inch.

From early spring to late summer, we sat on the cactus centered care home patio listening to gospel, old school R&B and Doo Wop. My heart soared when a familiar tune caused him to lift one foot. If he lifted both feet, I clapped like a grandparent at a kindergarten recital. Temptation was strong to leverage him to his feet and prop him up on the walker. My aching back and common sense overruled my heart. MH could not stand or walk without some measure of core strength, which he lacked.

As a passenger embarking on MH's Alzheimer's journey, I knew where we were going. It was hard to accept the destination. I stood back, attempted a subjective assessment of where we were at that time.

The runner slumped deep in the wheelchair never to walk again.

Physical therapists, caregivers and I tried our best to keep his wounded leg moving throughout the ordeal. Ironically, the left leg, which was not impacted by the surgery, took a bigger hit from inactivity than the right leg. The left leg went rigid, turned inward toward its wounded brother and led the race into atrophy.

The cheerleader in me refused to take "no" for an answer. With approval from his physical therapist, we continued to manipulate his legs with soft knee bends while he was on his back. The pillow between the knees did not provide enough resistance. I purchased a soft wedge to insert between his knees to separate his legs and prevent his big toes from overlapping.

The most prominent wound, extending ten inches down the outside of his leg had achieved some semblance of healing. It healed into a deep, disfiguring gulf, not at all cute. At least the pink and gnarly muscle tissue was no longer exposed.

Before the long-awaited healing a wound care nurse visited MH multiple times a week at the care home to uncover, clean and dress his wounds. It was like playing The Price Is Right. We never knew what was behind the curtain (or the bandages in this case). Too often there was a booby prize, a new eruption around the so-called "healing" wound, a weeping bedsore, oozing blood or mystery fluid. If this was a game, we were losing, big time.

The smaller wound on the inside of his leg turned out to be the granddaddy of them all. The nurses called it a "tunneling" wound due to its depth measuring eight centimeters at one point. When the wound care doctor probed as if searching for the bottom of a lake, I snatched away my eyes, silently swearing I would not subject my husband to torture without sedating him first. I did not care if he arrived at the wound doctor's office in a zombie like state. What the hell? He would not talk to them anyway. He groaned if the doctor hit a nerve. Who cared if he could not respond to their rhetorical question, "How're you doing today?"

"How do you think I'm doing with your gloved finger probing inside my leg?" I imagined MH saying.

Inability to sit up without support was an early indicator that MH's mind had wandered out to sea. MH could not sit unaided without collapsing. His left arm froze rigid to his body, tightly coiled, resistant to being extended. I truly believed that his ab muscles would kick in once we booted the viruses from his body, refined his diet and amped up his nutrition. Not so.

In bed MH was surrounded by a flotilla of pillows. Pillows were inserted under his knees to increase blood flow, behind his neck for support and on either side to allow rotation.

A couple of hours a day MH sat in a wheelchair chair with a pillow behind his head. He wore his ever-present compression boots that rested on top of an adjustable bench to prevent his feet from dangling without support. A small foam wedge was inserted underneath his left elbow and forearm to prevent him from leaning to one side. When I took him outside on the patio his props travelled with him.

Of all the symptoms of the rapidly progressing disease, the most annoying of all was his inability to smile. MH looked angry or unamused at all times. I tried explaining his expression to his three-year-old grandson. He heard the words but could not grasp why "Pops" did not seem happy to see him. I was sad that our grandson would never know the old Pops who could light up a room with his smile, dance with unabashed joy, give a fiery speech at a conference and sing "I Believe" from the bottom of his heart. The thief, Alzheimer's, had stolen that from us.

I asked MH's primary care physician to refer him, one more time, to a neurologist. I hoped the third time would be a charm. We entered the office of the same doctor who handed down the initial diagnosis. The encounter was radically different from before.

Dr. Pooni had mellowed substantially over the years. She sat close to the patient and addressed him directly, even though he was non-responsive. Seven years before she had stood over him, focusing on test results held stiffly in her hands. It proved that time and hundreds of close encounters with patients can smooth out the toughest physician and grant them a degree in humanity that outshines the diploma on the wall.

Despite her sweetened delivery, she remained no nonsense in her prognosis. My husband had reached Stage 6 of 7 on the F.A.S.T. scale.

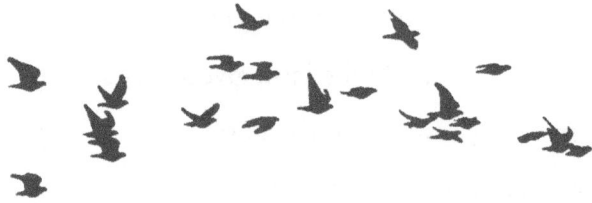

CHAPTER 16

AFTER THE FALL

We did everything possible to relax his muscles. This was an area where the occupational therapist, Leila, provided invaluable support. Leila had the magic touch. She demonstrated effective massage techniques for MH's back, shoulders and arms to relax tight muscles. She forced me to step up my game on providing MH with sensory stimulation to encourage his brain to work. Bring things from home that he relates to, Leila suggested.

MH's favorite sports figure was Muhammad Ali, the greatest boxer of all times. I framed a drawing of Ali (gifted to me by a friend) and posted it on his wall. I pointed to the wall, asked MH if he knew the man in the picture. MH mumbled, "Muhammed

Ali". Select long-term memory still existed. It needed coaxing to come out. My wheels were set in motion.

From the home that we had shared I brought more photo albums than he could read in a week. I surrounded him with family photos, remembrances of close friends from college and others who played important roles in his unfolding story.

None were more inspiring than Muhammad Ali. The coffee table book, *MUHAMMAD ALI* by Alan Goldstein contained a moving forward, written by George Foreman. MH loved the cover photo on the Goldstein book. The lipstick red of the title, Ali's glistening cherry red gloves, the animated ringside crowd on its feet mesmerized MH. Ali's flexed, brick hard biceps and open mouth towered above his dazed opponent, stretched out on the canvas. MH frequently flipped between the cover and the inside content, using his left hand, chronically glued to his left ribs, to hold down the book while turning pages with his right. The left hand that usually trembled like the epicenter of an earthquake, was eased into service by MH's hero, Muhammad Ali.

Muhammad Ali, A Thirty-Year Journey, by famed photographer Howard I. Bingham, was a testament to the bond between subject and photographer. A serene black and white photo of Ali in repose captured the depth of the champ's soul, beyond the flash and crowd adulation.

MH devoured the books, turned pages slowly, but steadily,

scrutinizing each photo. I stacked the books and photo albums, previously stored inside his closet, on the dresser for him to see and touch frequently.

I was on a roll, scavenging for familiar objects from MH's distant past. An oversized, vibrant Diego Rivera print of people dancing gaily in a plaza replaced a muted ocean view that ended in a solitary pier.

In life before Alzheimer's MH played solitaire. On a whim I placed a deck of cards in front of him. He arranged the cards by suit and in numerical sequence, using both hands, a physical and mental feat. It touched my heart to see him accomplish little tasks. For me his accomplishments were huge.

The tools employed to stimulate MH's senses (playing cards, dominoes, puzzles, books) may seem elementary. Those tools were essential to bringing MH's focus back to the center of the ring.

Physical and occupational therapy were helpful. Unfortunately, each round only lasted a few sessions. I learned to play the inside game. Additional rounds of physical and occupational therapy could be requested if I convinced the doctor that, based on the patient's progress, additional therapy was warranted. Persistence and patience were the keys to unlocking resources hidden behind closed doors.

Therapists could only help if the mind was able to process their instructions. When the cognitive understanding diminished to a certain level, there was nowhere else for the therapists to go. I groveled for every ounce of support he was eligible to receive.

My husband, the patient, was not always a star pupil. When the physical therapist arrived, MH refused to do the modest leg lifts he had done for me in private. He was like the kid who cried onstage at the Christmas pageant, even though he danced and sang like Sammy Davis at home in the living room. I rubbed his back, reassured him after each therapy session "you did great". I encouraged him, which encouraged me to find new ways to stimulate his brain.

On rare occasions MH's performance was nothing short of amazing. He held prolonged eye contact, spoke a series of intelligible sentences, matched dominoes, wrote his name better than he did before the Incident. Amazing days did not frequently repeat themselves. Amazing days were brain flares, shooting hope to the sky and to me. Everything else was predictable slog, no news being good news. Any day devoid of a trip to ER I considered a blessed day.

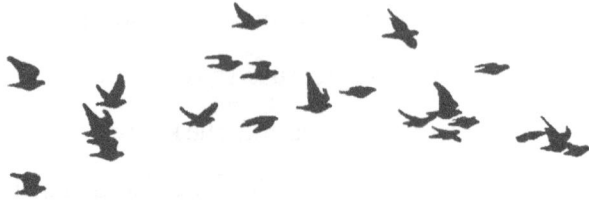

CHAPTER 17

A BLAZING GRACE

At an awkward time in the journey, it became tough to say, "I'm fine," when well-meaning people asked how I was doing. Awkward because MH was in a period of relative stability. He settled into his routine with no worrisome new wounds. There were no prescriptions for me to fetch, no undone assignments from therapists. All I had to do was stay on the treadmill of duties that became my routine and wait with the grace of a dutiful wife.

On the outside everything was calm, everything was light. Inside there was turmoil, volcanic fire burning to get on with my so-called life.

At three o'clock in the morning my eyes sprung open. Tired

feet planted on cool hardwood floors. A streak of Holy Ghost fire shot through weary bones.

"I'm too weak to do this," I shouted at empty bathroom walls until my throat hurt. I flopped onto the toilet seat and released an angry howl. He must not hear me, I thought. I blew my nose, tried to force my tense body to rise. I was glued to my throne of despair. So, I settled in and allowed myself to cry for what felt like hours.

Hands intertwined, elbows resting on my knees, I chastised God. "This was supposed to be the best days of our lives. Now he's stuck." My anger spewed out.

I knew that come morning I would clean up my unholy act, iron out my face that felt pulverized by a meat mallet.

I was angry. Certain issues in our marital relationship would go unresolved. Ultimately, those issues did not matter. I could not question or argue with a man with Alzheimer's.

Alzheimer's re-ordered our relationship. We fell into an unnatural rhythm. I became his perfect woman, the one he adored whenever I entered his room, unless I had been AWOL, in which case he glowered. His illness forced me to release all resistance, to love him without condition.

We never left each other's side without exchanging "I Love You." Why did pure love wait for crisis to arrive? We had wasted precious time.

Hours into my spiritual tsunami I was released from the throne.

As daylight eclipsed darkness, I toddled to my bed, added a footnote to my prayers. "God, please let me have a few hours of sleep. I am exhausted."

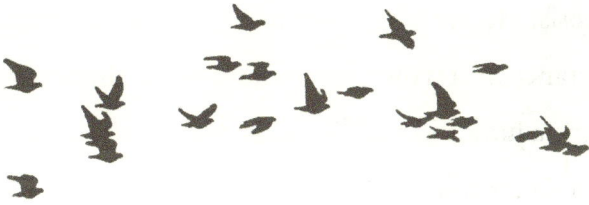

CHAPTER 18

APPETITE FOR ALZHEIMER'S

Throughout the course of his Alzheimer's journey MH's appetite took wild swings from food fetishes, fasting, binge eating to irrational restrictions on what he would eat. For months before the keys to the car were pried from his fingers, he consistently maintained multiple varieties of chocolate (brownies, cookies, candy) in the cupboard. The veneer on the hardwood pantry wore off from his repeated opening and closing. I tried hiding the sweets or throwing them away. Nothing worked. My husband simply returned to the store and purchased more. This chocolate fetish was bizarre for a man who had no special affection for chocolate pre-diagnosis. He, who sermonized to friends and relatives about the importance of staying in shape and maintaining good health, had become a junk food addict. Fortunately, the chocolate phase only lasted six months.

Not so brief was his love affair with fast food which lasted almost two years. MH consumed McDonald's for breakfast and Panda Express for lunch and dinner. Not only was this a blow to his fragile, inflamed digestive system, it was an insult to my culinary skills. Throughout our marriage I took pride in being a good cook. We ate dinner together regularly while seated at the table. Post diagnosis, I found myself eating alone or offering food to a man who turned up his nose at healthy food. I had to get over his rejection and find a way to stay sane.

Every morning MH demanded to be driven to McDonalds where he ordered his standard breakfast, which included coffee with artificial sweetener. No matter how much I carped about the danger of artificial sweeteners, Splenda it had to be. If I made a breakfast sandwich at home with fresh eggs and sausage, he looked as if my sandwich contained boo boo. Finally, I surrendered and let him eat whatever he wanted.

"Pull over," he insisted before we exited the McDonald's drive through. The brown paper sack had to be inspected to make sure he had everything. If anything, down to the black stirring stick, was missing from the bag I was commanded to run inside McDonald's, wearing a mask during the era of Covid-19, and correct his order.

Before Mickey D's was down the hatch, he insisted we stop at Panda Express to pick up a two item combo. Double order of sweet and sour chicken, one-half fried rice, one-half veggies, two containers of red sauce, and one chocolate chip cookie. The servers knew his order by heart. As soon as the Dodge pulled into the parking lot, they began preparing the order.

Occasionally, our timing would be off. We arrived at Panda Express ten minutes before the store opened at 11 a.m. We sat there counting minutes like the commercial where the people press their noses to the window and cry, "Open, open, open."

Was this fast food good for him? Of course not. MH harbored excess inflammation that could not be alleviated until he got his diet right. After losing battle after battle, I gave up arguing with a man in the throes of Alzheimer's about his diet.

For two excruciating years the Mac-Panda diet was engrained in his routine. At my urging, concerned friends and relatives tried unsuccessfully to talk him out of it. One good thing came out of the Incident. MH was cured of his fast-food addiction. During the time spent in the hospital MH seemed to detox. Massive doses of antibiotics could have done the job.

We were not sure what happened. The daily rides he demanded could no longer be accommodated due to his wounds. His appetite was curbed to the point that I became alarmed.

My worry about his fast-food consumption turned on its heels. The primary concern became, can he eat? Speech therapists tested him. The hospital would not feed him until they confirmed that he could eat without choking. Initially, I did not take the doctors and nurses' concerns too seriously. Of course he could eat, I thought, recalling all the Mac-Panda he consumed during the prior two years.

I rationalized that flavorless pureed food served in the hospital was enough to make anyone stop eating. I brought in and mashed up MH's favorite outside food, McDonald's and Panda Express. He toyed with it.

Ultimately, I was forced to accept reality. Something new had developed since his hospitalization. My husband had slipped into a later stage of Alzheimer's where chewing and swallowing became an issue. His ability to feed himself was marginal at best.

On release from the hospital to the board and care the doctor's orders did not restrict MH's diet. His mind seemed willing to eat, but there was no joy in it. MH voraciously crammed food into his mouth. Most of the food was "pocketed" in his jaws, not properly chewed or swallowed. Little food was being digested successfully. Clean-up was ugly. I dug chunks of chicken, steak and rice out of the mouth of a man intent on keeping his teeth clinched.

His weight plummeted.

I brought in softer foods, cottage cheese, yogurt, Ensure and Juven, different brands of high protein drinks. MH desperately needed protein to heal stubborn wounds.

In conversation with Haley, a wound care nurse who began visiting MH shortly after the Incident, she lamented the fact that, despite our best efforts, MH's wounds showed little improvement. I trusted her opinion. Haley was organized, caring, and took setbacks in his healing personally. Almost too personally. We comforted each other when MH's red, angry wounds leered as she unrolled layers of gauze from his leg.

Over time I found that the level of preparedness and profession-alism varied widely among nurses and therapists. Haley earned an "A" in both categories. She kept close contact with the wound care doctor's office, followed their instructions to the letter. I did not worry if I could not be on site at the time of Haley's visits, although I endeavored to be present any time a nurse or therapist entered my husband's room. I wanted their feedback, to see what they were seeing. I never fretted that Haley would miss a step or knowingly do anything to trigger a setback.

At the end of a particularly frustrating visit Haley commented, "Liquid protein is great, but in your husband's case it's not enough. There must be something more we can do."

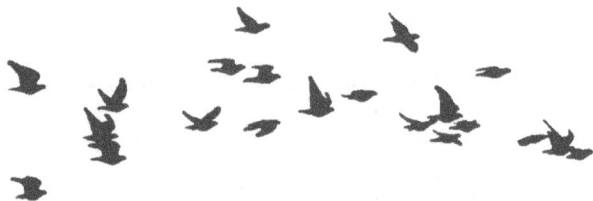

CHAPTER 19

BLENDER SPLENDOR

"More," became my rallying cry. Putting MH on a diet of flavorful, pureed food was a game changer. We fed him food he loved, but in pureed form. He ate, swallowed, and digested like a pro.

I started simply by modifying my sweet potato souffle recipe.

SWEET POTATO SOUFFLE

Ingredients:

6 medium sweet potatoes (deep red peel, orange inside)

1 cup milk (whole, low-fat, or almond)

3 tbsp. butter

1/4 cup sugar

1/2 tsp. vanilla flavoring

1/2 tsp. cinnamon

1/2 tsp. nutmeg

Pinch of salt

In a large pot boil whole sweet potatoes in 3 quarts of water until potatoes are soft when a fork is inserted. Use tongs to carefully remove potatoes from pot while they are still hot. Peel each potato and plop them whole into a food processor or blender. Add butter and mix until the butter is completely melted. Add sugar, vanilla, cinnamon, nutmeg, milk and a pinch of salt. Stir mixture until the flavor is evenly distributed. Taste mixture and make flavor adjustments as needed. If potatoes are naturally sweet or your loved one suffers from diabetes or high blood pressure, the sugar and/or salt may be eliminated altogether.

Serve warm. Hint: a dollop of whipped cream on warm souffle is great.

Sweet potato souffle was a game changer. He devoured real food that tasted good. Blending allowed him to swallow without gagging. The smooth texture eliminated "pocketing" of food. From that point forward we served him blended or pureed home cooked meals only.

I stored blended meals for my husband in sealed plastic containers purchased from the Dollar Store. Magic markers were used on masking tape to label the top. I specified the contents of each container (food was difficult to identify when blended) and the date prepared. If the food contained dairy or was quickly perishable, I included an expiration date.

When my mother was in the hospital after her final stroke, I spent more time at her bedside than at home in my own bed. My obsession with saving my mother did not help anyone. Thirty days into tinkering with "God's business" my mother succumbed to the inevitable. I was fifteen pounds lighter and looked like an anorexic in need of a chicken wing. My gaunt reflection in the mirror snapped me out of it. Sure, I wanted to lose a little weight like most middle-aged women with a pot gut. Allowing stress to take me down was not an intended or wise weight loss strategy.

I learned from hard experience that I could not help my loved one unless I stayed healthy. During my husband's journey I vowed to devote more time to taking care of me. Step one was cooking at home. I reserved a *pre-blended* portion of every meal for me to enjoy. That gave me readily accessible food to eat and no excuse to substitute a chocolate chip cookie for a meal.

For your convenience I have included additional recipes in Appendix A, which includes a recipe for chicken soup. With chicken soup on the menu my husband went from consuming very little real food to eating the equivalent of a full meal. I was ecstatic! I testified to everyone who had prayed for us and walked with us on this tedious journey. According to the doctors a time will come when my husband will not be able to eat at all. I made a conscious decision to do what I can, as long as I can. Tomorrow will take care of itself. Bon Appetit!

Beans featured prominently in my Blender Splendor meals. Number one, because of their high protein content they promoted healing. Second, they blended easily once they were cooked. Beans brought the taste and enjoyment of a home cooked meal to my loved one with impaired ability to chew and swallow. Bravo for beans, nature's wonder food.

My husband was blessed to have an excellent cook at the care home where he lived. My cooking frenzy was purely optional, intended to supplement the food he was already receiving. I coordinated with the cook to ensure that all his meals were pureed. It was useful to also share with my husband the tastes and seasonings that he enjoyed before Alzheimer's and before entering the board and care home.

Do not be afraid to make modifications. If the patient is intolerant to certain foods, eliminate them from the recipe or move on to a different recipe. In my husband's case, he thrived on getting the flavors he was accustomed to pre-Incident. Although blended, the taste was the same. I became sensitive to moderating the spices (e.g. using original rather than hot Rotel) to avoid choking.

I could not indulge my cooking binge until I sold the law practice that I enjoyed for many years. During the early days of my husband's diagnosis, the practice was not only financially rewarding, but emotionally sustaining. The practice allowed me to remove Alzheimer's, the Big A, from the headline of my day-to-day existence.

We were blessed to have our estate plan in order before the Big A hit. Fortunately, my law practice concentrated in the area of estate planning. We had in place our living trust, wills, durable powers of attorney and advance healthcare directives. MH's advance healthcare directive was handed to the hospital upon his admission. Being able to concentrate on MH's health instead of legal matters made a world of difference.

Ultimately, I reached the point where I could not keep all the balls in the air. I made a hard decision. I sold my practice to concentrate on what was most important to me. Family.

Keeping Alzheimer's from strangling our existence was essential. I use the term "us" consciously. Alzheimer's impacts the entire family. Loved ones caring for Alzheimer's patients are concerned about their own survival as well as the patient's. Statistics show that caring for an Alzheimer's patient significantly increases the risk of illness or death for the family caregiver. Neglecting to eat, to take care of personal health, exercise, sleep or engage in outside activities are bad habits that will mow down a caregiver quickly.

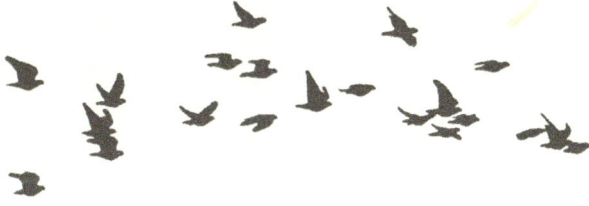

CHAPTER 20

FEAR OF HOPE

During this tedious, Alzheimer's journey I developed a chronic stealth condition which defied diagnosis. I now refer to it as "Fear of Hope". Dizzying ups and downs, heart clinching visits to ER and frequent doctor's appointments created negative expectations. Any minute either one of us would drown. I could not plan a long trip and if I left town for a brief respite, my traveling companion was always fear.

Planning became less exhausting after moving my husband into a board and care home where I knew he would be properly fed and kept clean. Still, my greatest fear was that the moment I boarded the plane something would happen to him.

The worst of times overlapped the best of times when our first grandchild was born in 2016. She was such a joy. It bothered me that she might not get to know her grandfather at all. But she did. Our granddaughter developed an uncanny compassion, rarely seen in a child so young, toward him. At age five she visited him at the board and care home. He sat on the edge of the bed. Granddaughter hugged him around the waist, burrowed her head into his chest and held on until he knew he was loved.

After the visit she asked questions far beyond her years. "Why can't Pops sleep at home with us?" The question brought me to tears. "I can't take care of him by myself. He can't walk so I need a man to lift him from the bed, the toilet, and the couch."

Explaining my decision to my granddaughter made me feel lousy all over again. She had not seen me struggle and fail to lift him, did not experience my nightmare of finding MH floating face down in the pool. For five years from the date of his diagnosis I pieced together a care plan, using outside caregivers to watch over him. Sometimes the plan worked. Most of the time it didn't. MH's needs were constantly evolving. Dependable, competent caregivers were difficult to find and hard to keep.

Moving MH to the board and care was one of the hardest decisions I have ever made. For the first couple of weeks MH insisted that I take him home. Many times, my guilty mind wrestled with whether I had made the right decision. Each time I asked the simple question, "And do what?" Stay awake listening for the sound of his restless footsteps, or even worse, the thud of his body hitting the floor? How long could I endure the backbreaking battle of lifting him up once he was down?

Added to that was the economics of the situation. The cost of full-time in-home quality care was astronomical. Estimates ranged between twenty-five and thirty thousand dollars a month using licensed and insured agencies.

I conferred with our son and MH's sister before making the decision. The weight of the decision fell on me. A lot of time was spent explaining my decision to other people (the budget busting cost of full-time in-home care, physical limitations in "transferring" (moving) MH, the emotional toll of being a full-time caregiver).

I waited a month after board and care admission to bring MH back to our home for a visit. He was a stranger in his own home. Agitated and anxious he could not wait to get out of there. I knew I had made the right decision. Home to MH was now the place where he felt secure. It was not with me. That did not prevent me from wrestling with loneliness and the agony of being separated from a man I had lived with for over forty years.

The day I came home from work and found MH soiled from the waist down, sunk into the couch, unable to lift himself up or sink to the floor, I knew a change had to come. Still, it took over a year to make the move. Neither he nor I could bear it.

The Alzheimer's stamp was an open-ended visa. No one knew the end date. The range of possibilities was broad. When I asked his primary doctor how long, the doctor demurred. "I've seen patients last anywhere from two to twenty years."

I toyed with the notion that MH would be the exception, that he would live for twenty more years into his nineties, like both of his parents. If his decline kept pace with what we already experienced, would living into his nineties be best for him?

Along the journey I established an informal network of people to share my experience. I chose not to join a formal support group like the ones available through Alzheimer's Association. My small group of six developed organically. Three women I met at the gym. One man I knew from a church that I previously attended. The other guy was a high school friend, whose wife developed Alzheimer's long after my husband and died within the space of two years. In one-to-one meetings by phone or in person we shared our stories and encouraged each other to keep on pushing.

My gym buddy Cassie returned to Body Pump weightlifting class after a three-week absence. She trudged in stoic, lips set to work out without acknowledging her pain. Five minutes into the workout Cassie's dam of tears overflowed. Fifty years of marriage to her recently deceased husband could not be ignored. The story rolled from her lips like rain. Her husband's final days consisted of complete inability to swallow, intense agitation and rambling thoughts as he wrestled with his inevitable fate. My fear of hope could not be contained.

Cassie was a member of the group I referred to as The Platinum

Circle, women over sixty-five, working out, fighting to stay in the game. We only saw each other on Saturday mornings at eight, congregated in the far corner of the workout room. We had claimed the same space in the Body Pump class for at least five years. First to arrive would set up equipment for others in the Circle.

Tita had been "Pumping" for years before I joined the class. As the first member of the Platinum Circle, I anointed her Queen. She was sweet, super friendly, flitted around the gym like a butterfly, engaging anyone with a minute to chat. Her lean, fit body and flash of frizzy hair locked in a messy ponytail welcomed all new members, including me and Cassie. Half the time I had no clue what Tita was saying, which I attributed to her combination of staccato English and Southeast Asian heritage. She babbled above the propane injected music and sometimes beyond the instructor's order, "Pick up your bar." I did not mind missing a few "reps" before Tita blundered back to her spot, two spaces ahead of mine.

Before Cassie's husband reached the end of his Alzheimer's trail Cassie and I noticed that Tita was missing more than a few "reps". Each week Tita showed up later to class. When I started at the gym, Tita would be the first one there. Difficulty in picking up the weights, adjusting weights between sets, keeping up with the instructor, became more apparent each week. More than the natural aging process was slowing her down. She lost more time "dilly dallying" with her backpack, getting ready to assume "set" position, than she spent exercising.

The real shocker was Tita's dwindling flesh. She had always been thin, but her latest emaciated look took it to another level. Her thighs were so bony and bowed you could draw a circle between them. I had my suspicions but was afraid to share them. Tita approached me about a referral to a nutritionist. I exhaled an audible sigh of relief. All she needed was help with her diet, maybe an appetite stimulator, I conveniently concluded. Diet could be fixed.

Two weeks later, Tita asked for the nutritionist's phone number again. I texted the number a second time and a third time when she forgot that she already had it. During one of Tita's recurring absences Cassie and I broke the ice about our AWOL gym buddy. Cassie had spoken to Tita's daughter and the family was aware of what they and we had observed.

"Don't set up her equipment anymore," the daughter suggested. "We're trying to keep her from driving."

"Good luck with that," I groaned under my breath. It was déjà vu. My frantic attempts to keep my husband from driving replayed in my mind: Trailing MH through the parking lot at McDonald's, MH attacking Lo Jack with a hammer, chisel, and a saw. I was disgusted that another family had to deal with the same issues. Disgusted that Tita's condition accelerated from bad to worse.

No one said the Big A out loud. We all thought it. Tita's daughter did not share what was really happening. Maybe she did not know. Maybe I did not want to know why Tita abdicated the throne as Queen of the Platinum Circle.

One out of six. Statistics said that one out of six people would be impacted by Alzheimer's. I scanned faces of the hopeful people, working out, futilely trying to outrun the shadow of death.

I reached down, added weight to each end of the barbell. I picked up the heavy bar, hoisted it over my head in salute to the Queen of the Platinum Circle.

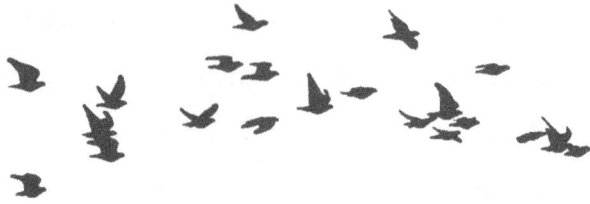

CHAPTER 21

LEANIN'

Every story was different. Each time there was a death within my loosely knit support group, my whole body clenched. Eventually it would be our turn in the center of the Circle. No matter how many pots of soup I stirred, it all came down to the truth confirmed at our first meeting with the Alzheimer's Association. Alzheimer's is a terminal disease.

Reliable research stated that MH's difficulty swallowing would morph into inability to swallow at all. Water and clear liquids were the greatest nemesis. If MH ingested too fast, hacking coughs racked his body. We quibbled over if and when to add thickener to the water. I tasted thickened water. Frankly, I would rather gag.

A sip of water every fifteen minutes was recommended by the

occupational therapist. Fine, when I was on duty. It was a tall order for in-house caregivers to follow. I wrestled with what to do. The answer remained the same. Do the best you can.

Desperate to know what went on inside his head, I read a ton of articles about amyloid plaques and tau tangles. AARP Magazine ran several informative articles on the subject. My binge reading provided little insight into his darkest moods, which I declined to label as depression or a bad case of the blues. Depression or the blues could lift with a change of circumstances. MH's circumstances were on a guaranteed downward trajectory. What he experienced was deeper than the blues.

Nothing explained how MH went from barely speaking for several months after the Incident to being more engaged, more aware of his surroundings as his wounds healed. I speculated that the absence of virus, pumping poison through his system, had a lot to do with it. As his nutrition improved his mood improved from mired in the certainty of sinking, to exercising a will to live. Sometimes I wondered if his resurgence was a cruel joke, setting me up for a crash landing, validating my fear of hope.

Was revival of MH's speech after months of silence cause for hope or just a teaser? One RN who treated MH shortly after the Incident stated that in a few cases patients recaptured a modicum of pre-Incident skills. First one, maybe two words came back, then on rare occasions complete sentences. When MH said, "I love you," "Kiss me", "Give me that", I got chills. During a long wait at a

doctor's office, he insisted repeatedly, "Take me back to the car."
He was not on the short list of replacement hosts for Jeopardy. The
fact that he communicated on any level felt like a miracle to me.

My faith was seriously tested. I was leanin' on the Lord to make
it day by day. I told myself that any amount of doubt about God's
ability to do the impossible was a sign of disbelief. In Philippians
4:6-7 the NIV Bible says: "Do not be anxious about anything,
but in every situation, by prayer and petition, with thanksgiving,
present your request to God. And the peace of God, which tran-
scends all understanding, will guard your hearts and your minds
in Christ Jesus."

Where does science end and faith begin? I turned to Bible buddies for help. Their prayers instantly lifted me up. For a minute.

In my worldly mind it was a game of basketball. One minute
I was up. Then the lead dwindled. The buzzer would sound. The
announcer would declare "Game Over". I could not keep it together
for more than a few minutes.

The specter of a loved one's death reminded me of my own mor-
tality. Multiply that by three (my father's death from Alzheimer's,
my mothers' loss from Dementia and my husband's looming
Alzheimer's) and you begin to ask serious questions, questions too
disturbing to raise in polite company. So I wrote it down on a Post
It. When the world empties of people we love, why are we still here?

Hardline so-called Christian fundamentalists will condemn me
as lacking faith. Concerned relatives might be tempted to commit

me to the looney bin for my own safety. Those who have walked in my shoes should rejoice. I found courage to ask the hard questions.

It was a full year after the Incident before I found the answer. We are here to marvel in our bountiful blessings, no matter how dire present circumstances appear. Our son and three grandchildren (a boy and girl were added as playmates and helpmates for our oldest granddaughter) are testaments to our blessings. God gave me a reasonable portion of health, sanity, and joy to journey with my husband through the Valley of Alzheimer's.

I set out to write a breezy, uplifting story of resilience. The more I wrote, my spirit pushed me to be real. Alzheimer's is a monster. Not the kind with rubber prosthesis, fake blood and pointy teeth. It is ethereal, untouchable and comes creeping in the night. There is no silver stake to drive through its heart.

Many times, I could not recognize my own life. Born into abject poverty I always found a way out. Alzheimer's was the most formidable foe I had ever met. It was ugly, rampant, indiscriminate, and never went to sleep. It stole the minds of lawyers, doctors, housewives, day laborers, pimps, sanitation workers and some who fall in multiple categories.

What held me down? Attending to my husband's needs, being able to serve left little time to question why the disease kept happening in my family. My friend sent a link to test for the likelihood of Alzheimer's. As of this writing, I have not taken the test. Am I afraid of the result? If the result was a high probability of Alzheimer's, every time I entered a room and could not remember why I was there, I would panic.

Serving was my consolation, the only peace I found. I recalled a sermon in which a prominent Southern California pastor admonished the congregation to quit whining about our loved one's sickness and start praising the Lord for giving us the health and strength to serve them.

I learned to count my blessings. I could not imagine the added anguish of the uninsured, unable to get treatment or afford pricey medications. When the pharmacist tendered a bill for four hundred and sixty-four dollars to fill one prescription, I turned into the roadrunner on speed. Mercifully, we had the resources to keep my husband above ground. Somewhere in this United States of America another human being lacked sufficient funds to get the medication they needed. Every time I walked out of the pharmacy, prescription filled, I thanked God.

Some people will complain that I bring faith into the discussion. For me faith and our walk through the Valley of Alzheimer's were inextricable. Without faith, rock solid or sometimes a tad bit shaky, we could not have stayed in the fight. Sometimes I did not know what to pray for. So, I simply asked God to walk with me through this journey as the primary caregiver of an Alzheimer's patient.

Recently I heard a sermon about leaning on faith in the time of struggle. The final point in the minister's three-point sermon was that struggle should not be a reason to lose faith. He spoke directly to my heart. The sermonic scripture was taken from Genesis 32:22-31, the story of Jacob, wrestling with God. Jacob refused to let go or surrender until God blessed him. I spent many days and nights camped out in hospital rooms, refusing to let go. As the shadow of death hung low, a gentle spirit whispered. Don't let go.

Listen to the doctor. Leave room for God.

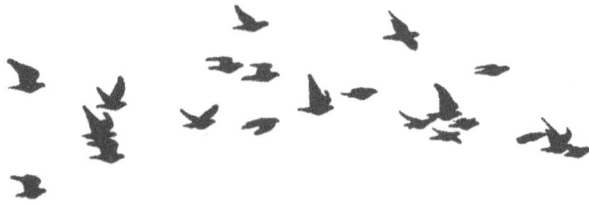

CHAPTER 22

FICKLE WILL FLEE

I recall a trip to South Africa three years before MH's official diagnosis. MH's inability to sleep on the seventeen-hour flight was a bummer. He paced up and down the aisles, which is normally a good thing on long flights. Anxiety bristled in his bones when I tried to calm him by rubbing his hands. Everything was "no" like a two-year old experiencing his first taste of power. By the time we reached the hotel in Johannesburg MH revved on all cylinders, too geeked to settle down. A travelling companion offered him sleeping pills. He grabbed the pills, greedily sucked one down. That night and every night to follow on our ten-day trip was a new revelation. He would sleep a couple of hours, then wander our room until he passed out. I slept with one eye open to prevent him from getting lost in a foreign country. One night the sleep bandit caught me bone tired, too exhausted to hear when he roused. I awakened to the trickle of urine hitting the front porch. I bolted from the bed, slipping and sliding through hot pee. With the door wide open, MH stood on the front porch, relieving himself.

"Who produces this much pee?" I thought.

In the blackness of night, the monkeys, giraffes, and zebras that strolled freely through the compound remained silent. The song of cicadas pierced the ink-stained night. I skidded to the restroom, the place where MH intended to be. I grabbed towels and soaked up a river of urine. I pulled him inside our room, stripped his wet clothes and eased him into the shower. His flat, unfocused stare convinced me that he was trapped between sleep and consciousness, even during the shower. The next morning, he remembered nothing.

At that point I discouraged MH from traveling alone. But traveling was in his blood. If I was unavailable for a trip, he insisted on going alone. I pleaded, "It's too dangerous." The only danger he perceived was in staying home. Alzheimer's intensified his urge to move. He aimed to outrun the disease that was gaining on him.

I missed traveling too. Travelling allowed us to be still, concentrate on each other, while exploring foreign places. I rationalized that the sleeping pills had caused the peeing episode. His reserved and limited interaction with our tour group I attributed to jet lag and the after-effects of sleeping pills. By sunset, soon after the evening meal, he would excuse himself and go to our room. I hung out solo with the rest of the tour group, making excuses for MH's absence.

On our trip to Bali, Indonesia my excuses did not hold water. We traveled with a group of close friends who had known MH for years. MH was hyper remote, unable to appreciate a joke or engage in friendly banter. His close friend of forty years asked bluntly, "What's the matter with my man?" I dropped all defenses, shared my unconfirmed suspicion. My man, who loved people, loved talking to anyone about anything, was on a solo journey into Alzheimer's.

Months later the unwelcome diagnosis dropped. My travel buddy was grounded. My couple card was pulled. Friends we had traveled with for years flew away as if Alzheimer's was contagious. In all fairness, some true friends tried to include us. But hanging around someone with Alzheimer's is not always fun. My husband transitioned from being the center of energy to being the center of scrutiny. People meant well, but they did not know how to handle it. Sometimes, neither did I.

I eliminated large gatherings from our calendar altogether. Too much stimulation pushed him deeper into a black hole. At small gatherings outside the home MH would eat and within minutes abruptly announce that he was ready to go. I gulped the contents of my red cup, grabbed my purse and we began the journey home. Bye-and-bye (as the old folks say) it became easier not to take him out at all. Our world shrank visibly by the day.

Except for a few friends that I will treasure forever, the invitations dried up. People were in a quandary, to invite or not to invite an Alzheimer's patient into a social setting. Would other guests be uncomfortable? There was no easy answer.

My neighbor explained that she had not visited my husband because she wanted to remember him "as he was". I understood her feelings, having witnessed human beings turn away from suffering or gawking at people who are less than perfect. My neighbor's response got me thinking. How often had I averted my eyes from a person afflicted with illness? Was I shielding the afflicted from the rudeness of my staring or shielding me from the reality that life can hurt.

At the early stages of the disease, I encouraged MH to participate as much as possible. He attended Bible Study at our home and was a part of every family function. As time went on, I was forced to become more vigilant about the activities he participated in. For example, I would not leave him alone to babysit the grandchildren when they visited. If he held a grandchild, I "spotted him" to make sure the child did not fall. MH had historically been the one who taught all visiting children to swim until I became concerned about safety. One moment of inattention could leave a lifetime of regret.

Certain activities, like movie going, he took himself out of. We were big movie buffs, enjoying movies at least twice a month. During one movie I was busy chomping on popcorn and cringing over blood and gore on the big screen. I glanced over at MH. He was on the verge of passing out. On screen violence, featuring Mickey Rourke as the aging, down and out boxer (cut, sweating and bleeding) was enough to make me shield my eyes from the screen. I felt Mickey's flabby flesh buckle with each blow, salty sweat leap into the audience from the screen. MH had chosen the movie. My preferred rom com could not move him from his slouch on the dreaded couch. To this day I do not know if MH's light headedness was caused by the on-screen violence.

I had pushed him too far, struggling in vain to maintain some semblance of a social life. In retrospect, that was selfish of me. His attention span had grown noticeably short. MH could no longer sit and focus on the big screen for two hours. We gave up on Friday night movies. We resorted to watching movies at home. Fifteen or twenty minutes in, he would quietly drift back to the bedroom and fall asleep. I quit rallying, "Babe, you're about to miss the good part," or running to the bedroom door, "John Legend is on stage." That stuff no longer mattered to him.

Branch by branch our social lives changed from vibrant green to brown before falling from the tree and withering. Walls of isolation closed in. We adjusted to our new normal. On days when I felt down, I beat back negative thoughts, reminded myself of what the preacher said. "I am blessed to be able to serve."

I pulled the Dodge into the brush free car wash line. The manager Paul looked at the car, then at me and beamed. His glistening teeth sparkled against skin the color of red clay. "How you doin?" Paul wrote the ticket without asking what I needed. We were regular customers for more than thirty years. "How's your husband?"

he asked as he did without fail every time I brought the Dodge in for a wash.

"I hope you don't mind me asking, but I think about him every time I see this car. He used to jump out, shadow boxing from the moment he got here. Then he'd take off down the trail. Said I reminded him of a fighter...I forget who it is. But anyway, tell him I asked about him."

I did not mind Paul asking about my husband at all. Caring people who remembered my husband could bring me out of whatever funk I was in. Caring people provided encouragement to keep walking down the trails that MH and I used to run. The Santa Ana riverbed trail, a bird and wildlife sanctuary, had been under construction for many years. Sadly, MH did not get to see the results of nature tamed by man. Water that stood stagnant for years now flowed into a graceful stream. The trail that was previously short and blocked by barriers now extended farther than I cared to walk. There was beauty above, in the hills of Anaheim, and below in tufted foliage. I inhaled the beauty of nature, winked at squirrels and wild rabbits zipping across the trail.

The days of MH's shadow boxing and running were over. Memories would live on in Paul and in the treasure chest of my heart.

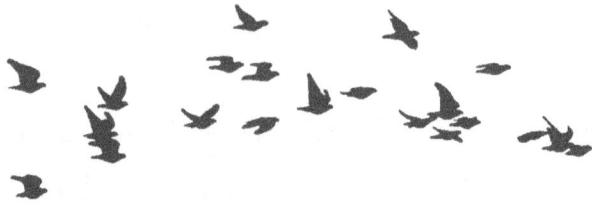

CHAPTER 23

LIGHT AT THE END

Every other day, wound care nurses washed MH's legs, injected Vashe wound solution into the openings, swabbed his cracked and bleeding heels with Iodine, stuffed the tunnelling wound with IODO Form Packing Strips, covered all wounds with pads and wrapped his leg in gauze.

At the end of the year wound care nurses declared the longest, branch like wound substantially healed. We were too exhausted to celebrate and too nervous about the tunnelling wound that remained open.

Friends reminded me that God moves in His own time. I saw no harm in reminding Him that we were still waiting for complete healing. I called in reinforcements, faithful Bible Buddies, people

I knew who could get a prayer through. I had resisted asking for prayer too often. Did not want to selfishly focus on my husband's needs. Other people were suffering, unchained chaos erupting in our land. I figured God was sick of hearing from me.

That night was special. I felt pushed to say what my husband needed. I asked my Bible Buddies to pray specifically for complete healing of MH's wounds.

Fervent, righteous prayer broke through the distance of ZOOM. The Holy Spirit took over the meeting that evening. I emptied out my worry, surrendered MH's healing into the arms of the Lord. Better than I had in months, I rested in perfect peace.

Fast forward three weeks. The visiting nurse informed me that the tunnelling wound had completely closed from the outside. The nurse was unable to pack it. His look of concern concerned me. The nurse said that it was unnatural that the tunnelling wound, recently measuring seven centimeters, had healed so quickly. Danger might lurk on the interior of the wound, according to the nurse. I listened as the nurse recited a list of negative possibilities. Had pockets formed inside the wound allowing infection to spread? If the wound was not completely healed from the inside, it might be necessary for the doctor to reopen it. The prospect of another surgery after a year of slow to no healing was more than I could conceive.

Subsequent wound care nurses were also amazed by the sudden closing of the tunnelling wound. They expressed the same concerns already pointed out to me. The only way to resolve the mystery was for the doctor to order a CT scan.

I channeled back to the point of surrender, refused to allow fear of hope to transform into desperate thinking. We had prayed specifically for wound healing and that is what we received. I acknowledged the blessing, gave thanks to my Bible Buddies.

On a cold day in November, we bundled up MH, muscled him into the seat of the Dodge and drove to the clinic for a CT scan of his leg.

Scars, running deep like a river, evidenced my husband's long, harrowing ordeal. CT test results revealed that MH's lingering wound had healed without evidence of infection. All praise belonged to God.

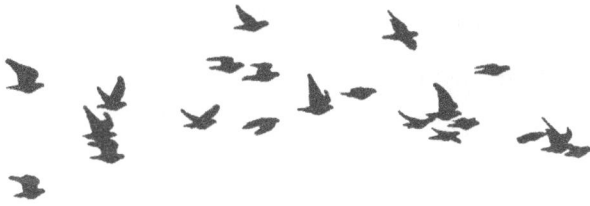

CHAPTER 24

DEEPER THAN BLUE

Back in the day, when his words flowed freely, MH frequently asked, "Take me for a ride." I knew exactly where he wanted to go: the Pacific Ocean that relaxed his knotted muscles and released his inner peace. To the ocean that corralled his rambling thoughts, running deeper than the blue his eyes could see.

The ocean caressed his body, metaphorically. My husband's feet never touched the sand. Each time I begged him to get out of the car, his answer was an unequivocal "No". MH sat in the Dodge and watched the ebb and flow of the tide, taking him farther and deeper out to sea. I quieted the music, let myself drift as far as he allowed me to go.

I could never reach that distant shore where his mind lingered. I could not barge beyond the limits of my ordered thinking.

At the ocean MH was free. Free from my questioning, "What are you thinking?" He was free from the inane probing of where his mind was as he sat right next to me. I craved a machine that could lead me to the place where his thoughts resided. When the silence settled in, I found myself pandering for his attention, asking out loud, "Is there something you want to tell me?"

Over time his words reduced to simple instructions, "Kiss me," "Give me that," "Take me inside the house," "Let's go." The "why's" became eternally unanswerable. Even if I asked, I would never know what he wanted me to do about his predicament, which was completely beyond my control.

As the years rolled by, I was greeted by his tears more frequently than my heart could bear. Watery eyes scrunched together his bushy brows. His lips scrolled away from his teeth. Tears flowed inexplicably. A remembered song from his distant past, a Sly Stone classic, would set him off. A photograph of his son or grandchildren could open the floodgates. I counted those as tears of joy. Other tears spelled pain, remembrances of moments no longer within his grasp.

I tamped down my tears to prevent our visits from becoming "pity" parties. I held his trembling hands in mine. My fear: MH was locked in a cage, submerged in deep water, struggling to get out. I banished the thought and subdued my panic. I prayed that the anti-anxiety meds would not let his mind go there, that I was only imagining his suffering. Whatever his state of mind, it was deeper than blue, as dark as the existence he held onto.

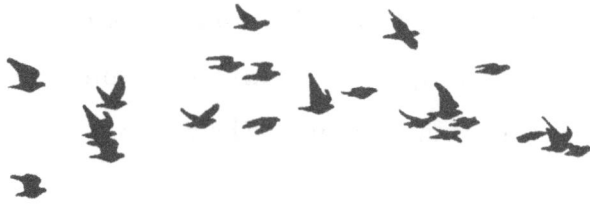

CHAPTER 25

WHAT THE END'S GON' BE

The race against Alzheimer's reminded me of the early 1980's when MH "hit the wall" less than a mile from the finish line of the Detroit Marathon. I was posted up near the end waiting for MH to appear on the horizon. An hour after his anticipated finish time I began to worry. Something had gone wrong.

In the distance I saw his gleaming white tank top, red shorts and red bandana floating like a mirage. His unsteady legs wobbled from side to side. MH's shoulders were down, his face ashen, drained of blood. His fingers unfurled like a dazed boxer. He refused to go down.

Without thinking I jumped into the jumble of runners, motley stragglers, clawing their way to the finish line. I could not touch MH, or he would be disqualified.

I walked alongside him while singing the Patty Austin and James Ingram version of "Baby, Come to Me". His caved in shoulders straightened a bit, feet steadied enough to trot in a forward direction. He stopped, staggered, and lifted his head. I sang louder until my hoarse voice was drowned out by "We Are the Champions" booming at the finish line.

MH exhaled his first deep breath since cresting the horizon. He pressed on.

My focus fell to his feet, fighting for every step. "Hold your head up, babe. You can do this!" I cheered him on, stepped back and faded into the pumped-up crowd.

MH crossed the finish line. Alone.

APPENDIX A

Chicken Soup

Ingredients:

3-4 chicken breasts

1 onion (chopped)

1 large potato (cubed)

4 cloves of garlic (chopped or crushed)

3 celery stalks

1 cup baby carrots (sliced)

6 oz. whole kernel corn (fresh or canned)

6 oz. can green beans (strained)

Two 10.5 oz. cans of cream of chicken or cream of celery soup

3 bay leaves

Salt and pepper to taste

Red pepper flakes to taste (optional)

Rinse and dry chicken breasts. Season with salt and pepper to taste.

In skillet brown seasoned chicken breasts in olive oil. Stir in onions when breasts are almost done. When onions are translucent add garlic and sliced celery for one minute.

Remove chicken breasts from skillet to a cutting board and chop into bite size pieces.

In a separate 6 qt. pot warm both cans of soup. Stir frequently. When the soup is warm, but not boiling, pour water into empty soup cans and slowly add to soup base. Increase heat, but do not boil. Add chicken mixture to the pot. Add potatoes, carrots and bay leaves to the pot. Add salt, pepper and crushed red pepper, if desired. Go easy on the pepper, which may cause coughing or gagging.

Cook on low heat for approximately twenty minutes or until the carrots and potatoes are done. Add corn and green beans for the last ten minutes. Puree in blender or food processor.

White Bean Soup

16 oz. package dry Great Northern Beans

14.5 oz. can Mexican style stewed tomatoes

2 smoked turkey legs or wings

6 cloves garlic (chopped or crushed)

Medium sweet onion (chopped)

1 tsp. seasoned salt

½ tsp. white pepper

½ tsp. garlic powder

½ tsp. onion powder

½ tsp. crushed red pepper (optional)

2 bay leaves

½ tsp Louisiana hot sauce

1 tbs. golden brown sugar

1 tbs. olive oil

Open package of beans, sift through to eliminate any naturally occurring pebbles. Rinse beans at least twice. Cover beans with water and allow them to soak for one hour.

Rinse turkey parts and boil in 3 quarts of water for ½ hour with lid on pot. In separate pan sauté onion in olive oil for approximately one minute. Add hot sauce and garlic and sauté for approximately 30 seconds. Add sauteed mixture to boiling turkey parts. Cover pot and simmer contents for one-half hour.

Drain water from beans and add beans to pot with turkey parts. Add stewed tomatoes, all remaining seasonings and sugar. Stir, bring to a boil. Reduce heat and simmer for the greater of one hour or until the beans are softened, intact, but not crunchy. Puree in blender or food processor.

Taco Soup

2 lbs. ground turkey

2 -16 oz. cans pinto beans

1-16 oz. can of Rotel (original)

1-16 oz. can Mexican style diced tomatoes

1 large, sweet onion, chopped

4-6 cloves garlic, chopped or pressed

1/2 tsp. salt

1/2 tsp. pepper

2-1 oz. pkgs. taco seasoning mix

4 oz. whole kernel corn

1 oz. package of ranch seasoning (optional)

Mexican four cheese blend (farm style shreds, if available)

Fresh cilantro (optional)

Sprinkle salt and pepper over ground turkey. Brown in medium skillet. Add ½ package of taco seasoning mix to meat.

In separate small skillet sauté onions until onion is translucent. Stir in garlic for one minute.

In a separate large pot combine Rotel, diced tomatoes, pinto beans and corn. Cook on medium heat for five minutes. Slowly add the remaining one-half package of taco seasoning. Add meat, onion and garlic from skillet to the large pot. You may add one-half package of ranch seasoning, stirring constantly, if desired. (Note: you will save ½ package of ranch seasoning for another meal). Reduce heat. Simmer for fifteen minutes to blend flavors. Individual ingredients are already fully cooked. Puree in blender or food processor.

Garnish: On your personal, pre-blended serving sprinkle Mexican four cheese blend, fresh cilantro and low sodium Fritos corn chip. Do not make a habit of adding Frito's to your personal serving but try it at least once. Your taste buds will thank me.

Black Bean Soup

16 oz. package of dried black beans

1 large smoked turkey leg or two turkey wings

1 large onion-chopped

6 cloves of garlic-chopped

2 stalks celery-veins removed and sliced

½ to 1 tbs. cumin

1 tsp. salt

½ tsp. red pepper flakes

1 tbs. fresh lime juice

¼ cup fresh cilantro (optional)

Avocado (optional)

Sour cream (optional)

Sift through dry beans to eliminate any naturally occurring pebbles. Rinse beans two to three times. Cover beans with warm water and allow them to soak for one hour.

In large 6-quart pot boil turkey leg with one-third pot of water and bring to a boil. In a small skillet sauté onions until translucent. Add garlic and celery and continue to sauté for one minute. Add sauteed garlic, celery and onion to large pot. Cook on medium heat covered for one-half hour.

Drain beans and add to large pot. Water should cover the beans and turkey leg. Add cumin, salt, pepper, red pepper flakes and lime juice and bring to a boil. Lower heat to medium. Cook for approximately forty-five minutes to an hour or until beans are done. The beans should still be intact, but not crunchy. Juice of the beans should be slightly thickened, like a thin gravy. Puree in blender or food processor.

Brussel Sprouts

1 lb. fresh Brussel sprouts

1 tbs. butter

Steam Brussel sprouts for five minutes after water comes to a boil. Melt butter over Brussel sprouts while warm. Puree in blender or food processor.

Note: In lieu of Brussel sprouts you may use carrots, broccoli or cauliflower. Reserve water beneath the steamer in case you need to add liquid to pureed vegetables.

ABOUT THE AUTHOR

AMANDA G. IS THE AUTHOR of three published novels. Two of her novels, *Arms of the Magnolia* and *Beyond the Fire*, were published by Fawcett Books. Her recent novel, *Confliction*, published by GW Publishing LLC, was her first edge-of-your-seat suspense thriller.

Deeper Than Blue is Amanda G.'s debut in non-fiction. "Something deep within my spirit compelled me to write the story I was witnessing on a day-to-day basis, my husband's journey through the valley of Alzheimer's. I pray that someone will be lifted by sharing our experiences."

Amanda G., a graduate of the University of California, Berkeley, School of Law, is a retired estate planning attorney.

www.ingramcontent.com/pod-product-compliance
Lightning Source LLC
Chambersburg PA
CBHW031129020426
42333CB00012B/294